MW00352138

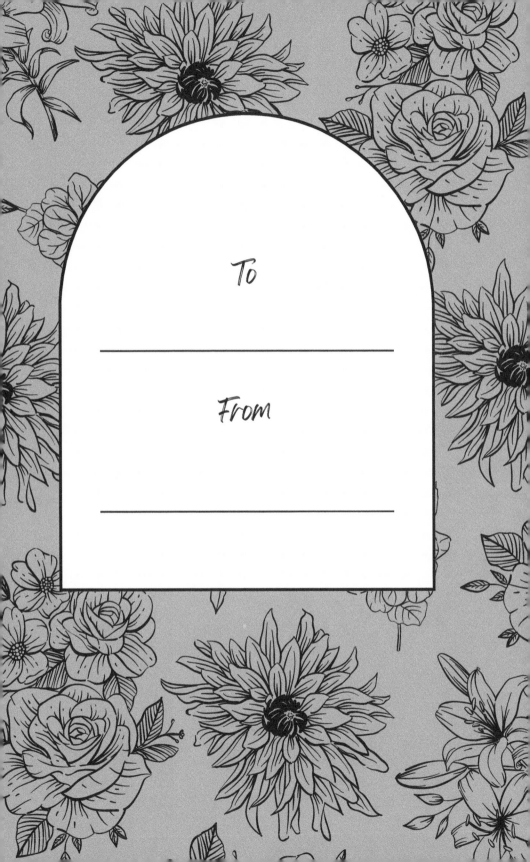

To

_____

From

Endorsements

"What a precious and beautiful book, inside and out. Torrie's words pulled me in so much that I felt as if I could feel her longing and her suffering myself as if I was feeling so deeply for a dear friend. Her words of faith will stretch you, comfort you, and you wilL want to soak up every word of this book."
-Dawn Barton
(Author, Speaker, Joyologist)

"I am so proud of Torrie for dreaming big and sharing her story. She is a bright light! Let her story of redemption give you hope that God will bring beauty from pain and joy from sorrow."
- Britt Nicole
(Recording Artist, Songwriter, Dove Award Winner & Grammy Nominee)

"What a wonderful account of God's faithfulness through the trials of life! Torrie's stories are so relatable to anyone walking through the ups and downs of life. As I read through each account of Torrie's own personal journey, I could sense the emotion of the experience. No matter where you are in life, this is a great book to add to your reading list.
- Marty Payton, DMin
(My Pastor, Charity Baptist Church, Kannapolis, NC)

"The longing is the bridge that connects a woman who desires to bear children, to the promise of God's love and plan for her life."
-Melissa Lynn Hunt
(Founder & Visionary Genuine Teams, Editor-in-Chief for Genuine Magazine)

The
Longing

A relatable journey to motherhood, through
infertility and miscarriage while finding
God's promises along the way.

Torrie Jarrett

UNITED 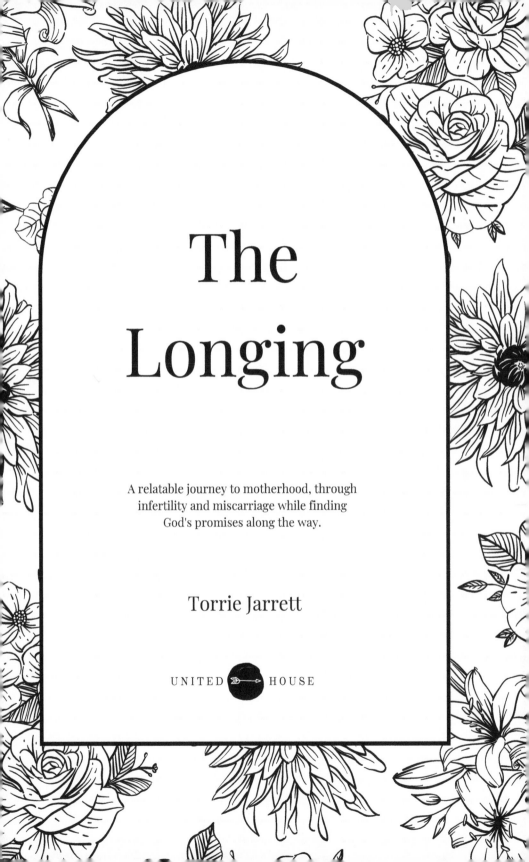 HOUSE

Scripture marked (NLT) are taken from the Holy Bible, New Living Translation, copyright © 1996, 2004, 2015 by Tyndale House Foundation. Used by permission of Tyndale House
Publishers, Inc., Carol Stream, Illinois 60188. All rights reserved.

Scriptures marked (ESV) are from The ESV® Bible (The Holy Bible, English Standard Version®), copyright © 2001 by Crossway, a publishing ministry of Good News Publishers. Used by permission. All rights reserved.

Scriptures marked (NIV) are from THE HOLY BIBLE, NEW INTERNATIONAL VERSION® NIV® Copyright © 1973, 1978, 1984 by International Bible Society® Used by permission. All rights reserved worldwide.

Scripture quotations marked MSG are taken from The Message, copyright © 1993, 2002, 2018 by Eugene H. Peterson. Used by permission of NavPress. All rights reserved. Represented by Tyndale House Publishers.

New American Standard Bible®, Copyright © 1960, 1971, 1977, 1995 by The Lockman Foundation. All rights reserved.

Scripture taken from the New King James Version®. Copyright © 1982 by Thomas Nelson. Used by permission. All rights reserved.

ISBN: 978-1-952840-34-0

UNITED HOUSE Publishing
Waterford, Michigan
info@unitedhousepublishing.com
www.unitedhousepublishing.com

Cover and Interior Graphics: Torrie Jarrett
Interior Formatting: Matt Russell, Marketing Image, mrussell@marketing-image.com

Printed in the United States of America
2023—First Edition

SPECIAL SALES
Most UNITED HOUSE books are available at special quantity discounts when purchased in bulk by corporations, organizations, and special-interest groups. For information, please e-mail orders@ unitedhousepublishing.com.

Thank you for picking up this book. Thank you for opening it to reveal the beautiful message that God has delivered. He is with us through every desire and longing of our heart. He utterly love us, His children and He wants to create an unshakable relationship with us through this difficult journey we call life. I'm sending a hug and lots of love to comfort you during whatever season of longing you might be living in as you read the pages of this book.

xoxo, Torrie

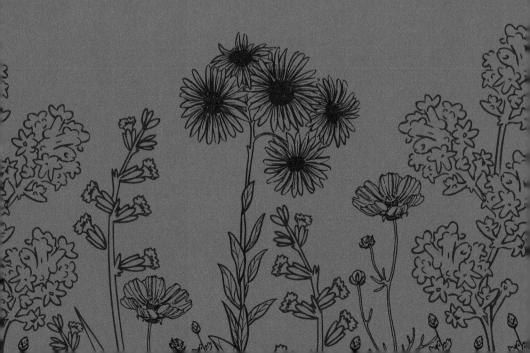

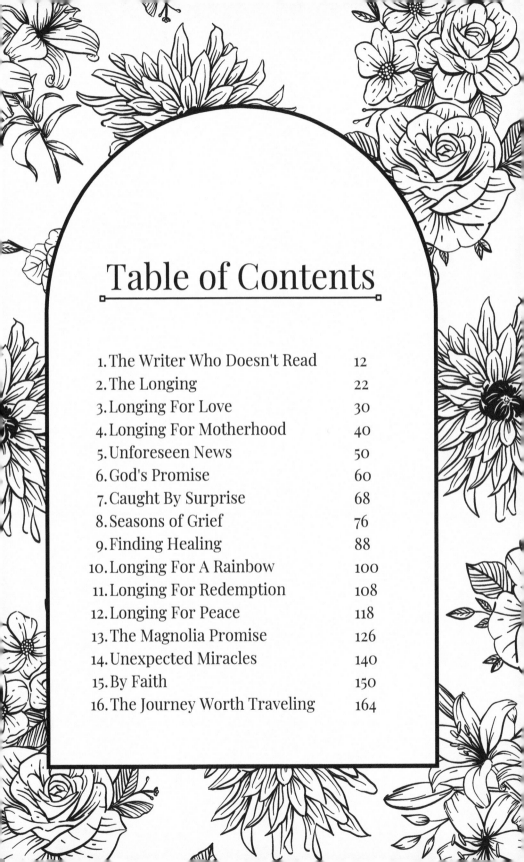

Table of Contents

Chapter 1

The Writer Who Doesn't Read

Each of you should use whatever gift you have received to serve others, as faithful stewards of God's grace in its various forms. If anyone speaks, they should do so as one who speaks the very words of God. If anyone serves, they should do so with the strength God provides, so that in all things God may be praised through Jesus Christ. To Him be the power and glory forever. Amen.

1 Peter 4:10,11 NIV

Each of you should use whatever gift you have received to serve others, as faithful stewards of God's grace in its various forms. If anyone speaks, they should do so as one who speaks the very Words of God. If anyone serves, they should do so with the strength God provides, so that in all things God may be praised Through Jesus Christ. To Him be the power and glory forever. Amen.
1 Peter 4:10 & 11, NIV

I have a little secret … Are you ready for it? It's a pretty big one … Okay, don't judge me, but I don't really love to read. *AHHHH!* Embarrassing, right? I mean, I love the idea of reading and the feeling of a book in my hands, but I just really struggle to channel my thoughts when I crack open a book. I have bought many books over the years. I adore them, actually, and I'm a sucker for books with a good cover. Yes, I admit it. I judge a book by the cover, breaking the one rule given over and over by every teacher in the history of teachers: DON'T JUDGE A BOOK BY THE COVER. But truthfully, if the author could capture my attention for any length of time, or has anything in common with something I would like to read, the cover must be appealing, right? And, right about now, on the very first page of my very first book, you are closing it to examine the cover closely, right? Yikes. I hope it's a good one. Foot in mouth on page one. Yup, that's me. I always speak things before I fully think about them, and then I ponder on how l could have worded things differently for hours thereafter.

So, since my foot is already in my mouth, let me just go ahead and lay the rest out there for you before you get an image of me as an AUTHOR (insert glowing lights from the ceiling). I'm a human. Hi! It's me, Torrie Jarrett, the human who says the wrong things, judges books by their covers, goes a little too far to make someone laugh, sometimes gets upset at the tiny things, cries

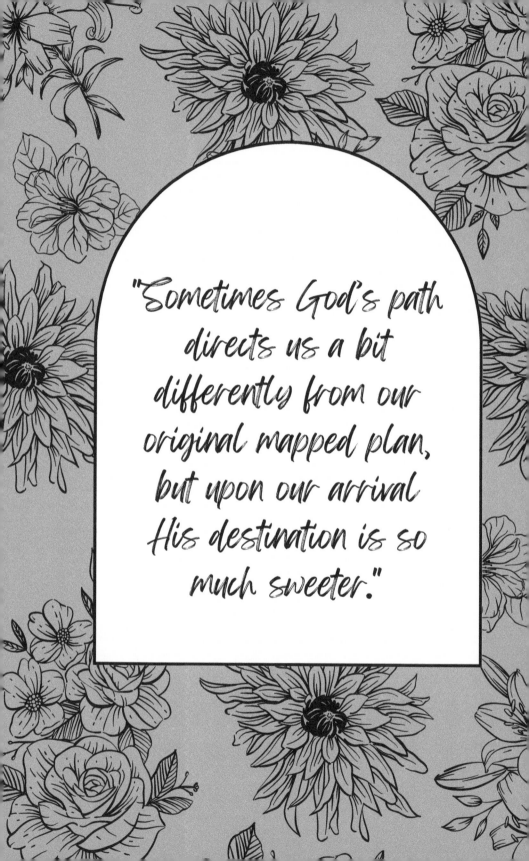

"Sometimes God's path directs us a bit differently from our original mapped plan, but upon our arrival His destination is so much sweeter."

at Folgers commercials (every time), forgets friends' birthdays, has forty-five unanswered texts in my phone at any given moment, and are you ready for it ... DOES NOT READ!! Eh, yeah, I said it. I wrote a book, keep a blog, home-school my kids, and I simply just struggle to keep my thoughts in line enough to read a book from cover to cover. In fact, I have only read a few complete books in my adult life (or any stage of my life). However, if you walk into my house, you will find books in every corner. I have shelves filled with them. I have books on the coffee table, mantle, setting on end tables, dressers, and nightstands. They are comforting to me. I love buying books. I make my kids read daily, and if you hired me to decorate your home, I would bring stacks of vintage books of all colors and fill your shelves with them. But, when I sit down to read a book it goes a little like this ... once upon a time, (squirrel), there was a lovely young girl (did I switch over the laundry?), and she lived in a (what line was I on again, oh lovely), lovely young girl, and she lived (oh my gosh, I forgot to respond to Lauren, I better do that before I friend-fail again ... Wait, where's my phone?) ... You see how it goes? My thoughts race faster than an Arabian racehorse, and taming my mind is a task I work very hard at daily.

So, if you're wondering at this point, why does this girl write but doesn't read, I have no answer to that. I actually never knew it was a thing until I heard other authors have this same battle as well. Actually, the very reason I have never sat down to write a book is that, several years ago, I felt God calling me to do so. So, I talked to a close friend and told her I have a new five-year plan, and I am going to write a book. Her response was: "How are you going to write a book? You don't even read them." It captivated me, and I believed her words were true. So, what did I do? I bought books. Mom books, marriage books, devotionals, Bibles, and even books on friendships. I bought them all, and every time I didn't finish one, the words echoed in my ear. *Failure, ridiculous-ness, never going to meet your goals*, and so on. Until one day, I read the words from another author, "You don't have to be a reader to be a writer."[1] I couldn't believe it, actually. I had lived by the words "you must read to write" for so long, and now I was released from the bondage that held me under. When I freed myself from the lies I had been living, I was fully able to hear God's voice speaking over my life, and this is what He was saying: "It's time! It's time for you to tell your story. You don't have to read books to write a story I created specifically for you. Tell the world about me and the magnificent ways I have worked miracles in your life." Friend, it was literally at that moment, I wrote down the table of contents of this book you now hold in your hands. A year prior to this encounter, God told me the title would be *The Longing*, but I just figured I would be worthy to write it when I turned fifty or older, because after all, most fifty-year-olds like to read, right?? (See, foot in mouth!)

So, now that I've given you my dark secret, let's really get to know each other. If you still aren't convinced I am just as human as you are, let me just go ahead, before we finish this chapter, and open up my closet door. My resume of perfection ends here, I assure you. I have never spoken at a conference, I'm not famous, I live in a small town, and I am a mother of four children who often loses her temper and regrets it immediately after. I have lost two babies (which I have a hard time not adding to the number of children I have when people ask). We have been homeschooling for four years, and most days, I feel like I live on a struggle bus, but I push through and give each day the best I can. I have been a cosmetologist for seventeen years but decided I needed a career change and switched paths to home design about five years ago. I'm married to a contractor, and we own Willowbrook Builders, doing anything from bathroom remodels, whole house renovations, and new home builds. And, as if that wasn't enough to fill up my days, we recently opened a little coffee shop in the small town of Landis, NC.

Whew!! So, now that I have covered all of my recent events, let's get a little deeper into my closet where the really dusty parts dwell. I grew up in a very small church, in a little mountain town, as the pastor's daughter. Being the pastor's daughter held me to a higher standard, and on most days, reminded me there was no room for flaws in the day-to-day choices and actions I made. Perfection was something I strived for daily as I allowed the opinions of others to place substantial value on my life. Thankfully, God doesn't examine us this way, and now I realize HE is the only one capable of living a perfectly spotless life. Unfortunately, this was a lesson that took me many years to grasp.

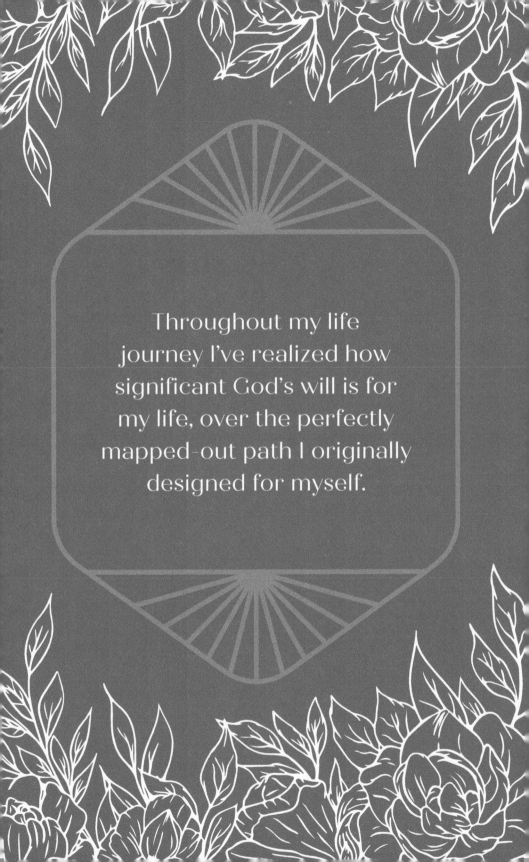

Throughout my life journey I've realized how significant God's will is for my life, over the perfectly mapped-out path I originally designed for myself.

Never be afraid to do the thing God is equipping you to do.

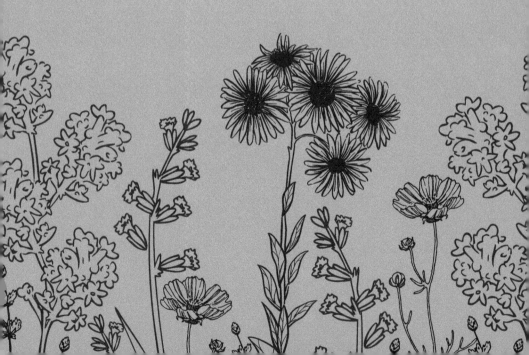

Throughout my teen years, I held onto the biggest dreams of becoming an entrepreneur and owning multiple businesses. You could blame these ambitions on my God-given Enneagram[2] type seven personality and internal fear of missing out on something amazing. My life intention list consisted of owning a salon, coffee shop, and working in fashion design, all the while being a wife and mother of four kids. If you're wondering if this list is attainable, it would be a great time for me to announce, "With God, ALL things can be POSSIBLE, as long as it's HIS will for your life." Sometimes, God's path directs us a bit differently from our original mapped plan, but upon our arrival, His destination is so much sweeter.

Okay, so now that the closet has been sorted, and we have become friends ... I think we can get on with this book, don't you?

This book will take you through some of my life journeys, and I will share God's unconditional love as He revealed it to me throughout His promises on my life. Many years of my life have been engulfed by the deepest longings, longing for love, motherhood, a home, farmland, and business ownership. Throughout my journey, I have experienced losses, failures, and unexpected turns. These losses immensely magnified the longing I had within, but throughout my emotional excursion, I ultimately found the presence of God, and my faith grew exceedingly. My hope for you in reading this book is that you will experience the embrace of God's love covering you during an hour of longing. I pray your eyes are opened to God's capability to arrive in the darkest moments of your life with the most unforeseen, perfect timing. It was during these seasons of life when I realized how deeply He longed for me the way I longed for my dreams (husband, babies, farmland, etc.).

Throughout my life journey, I've realized how significant God's will is for my life, over the perfectly mapped-out path I originally designed for myself.

If you have picked up this book, you must be longing for something, and I want to let you know, YOU ARE NOT ALONE. This journey through life is an extremely difficult adventure, but God's presence is all around us. He has a significant plan for your future and the most impeccable timing, which is so much better than our own.

Your longings will be fulfilled, but they might not be in the specific order you planned them or the exact process you had in mind.

And that, friends, will be okay, too.

Chapter 2

The Longing

> My soul longs, yes, faints for the counts of the Lord; my heart and flesh sing for joy to the living God.
>
> Psalm 84:2, ESV

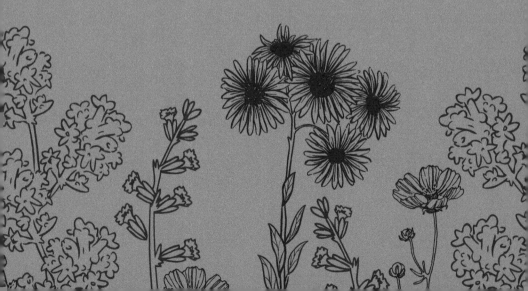

My soul longs, yes, faints for the courts of the Lord;
my heart and flesh sing for joy to the living God.
Psalm 84:2, ESV

What does longing for something actually mean? I have *wanted* many things. I have *wanted* to be taller my entire life. I'm 5'2", and life on the lower level hasn't always been the greatest thing. Every pair of pants I buy must be hemmed (thank the Lord for frayed hems becoming a thing these days). Unfortunately, my toes will one day look like my dear ol' Nanny's did, crawling all over each other, because this girl chooses to wear a heel with pretty much every outfit. Shelves must be climbed at the grocery store every time I need pimentos (I make a mean pimento cheese) and getting into my husband's jacked-up truck, in a dress, while the wind is blowing on Sunday morning ... Well, let's just say it doesn't come easy, and please don't stand behind me.

So, would you say these are longings? For me, the answer would be no. This is who I am, and though, sure, I would love a little growth spurt in my thirties, it's not something I long for. And I haven't grown since the fifth grade, so I've become pretty accustomed to my height. Now, if you want to talk about arms, I would definitely put that in the longing category. I am a rather petite person with an athletic build and throw in a little cottage cheese here or there if ya will (hello, mom of four kids, no one's perfect). These arms I have were inherited straight from my Nanny and have so graciously been handed down from generation to generation. I have done pretty much every arm workout there is, and these babies just don't slim down. Now, don't get the idea I spend a lot of time in the gym. I am a faithful January gym rat. I work out enough in January to cover the entire year (can I get an amen??). I gave up wasting my New Year's resolution on getting in shape for the beach years ago. Instead, I began setting an attainable goal ... work out the month of January and be done! Now, that's

long·ing

/'lôNGiNG/

noun

a strong desire
(esp. for something unattainable).

Webster Dictionary

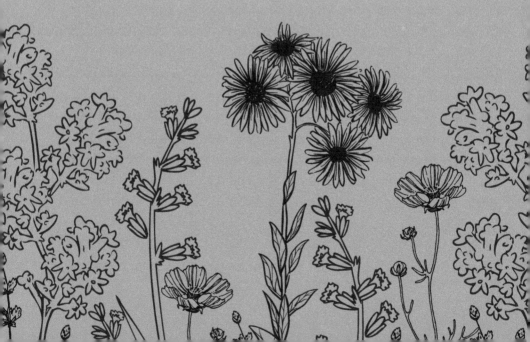

a resolution I can keep.

So, when I say *the longing*, what is the first idea that comes to mind for you? Is there a life you see yourself living, a new home you wish to reside in, or a career you hope to obtain? Do you dream of becoming a mother, rocking babies, and living your life as a family of four? Or, do you wish your marriage was Instagram fabulous and your relationship more resembled a romantic scene from a Hallmark movie?

For me, longing has been that deep, pit-in-your-stomach feeling, when you want something so badly it hurts. It's that profound desire that keeps you awake at night praying for God's fulfillment.

Merriam-Webster's definition of *longing* is a strong desire[3]
(esp. for something unattainable).

That's it. Such a small definition for one of the most profound words, don't you think? A strong desire for something you want but feel like may never happen. I can recall many longings in my life over the years, and I share them with you throughout the chapters in this book. I have laid awake many nights begging for God to answer my prayers and have also taken a drive for many extra miles in my car, singing at the top of my lungs, while praying for miracles to happen. In fact, (side note) most of my prayer time and focus were obtained in long car rides. I love to ride with the windows down, the sunroof open, oversized sunglasses on my face, worship music loud, and my favorite coffee in hand.

One of the first longings I can remember as a child was for a Cabbage Patch Doll. I lost a lot of sleep over that doll because I had somehow forgotten to ask for it when I went to visit Santa Claus. You could blame it on my nervousness or the fact that the entire time I sat on his lap, I just wanted to yank his beard to see if it was real or not, but I totally forgot to ask him. I was five years old at the time, and in my childlike mind, this was an utter disaster. I just knew on Christmas morning the doll wouldn't be there. I mailed a letter to the North Pole, I prayed to God asking for a tiny miracle, I told my parents over and over needed that doll, and on Christmas Eve, I left a note beside the milk and cookies that read like this:

> Dear Santa,
> I really want a Cabbage Patch Doll, but I forgot to ask you for one. If you have an extra one in your sack, will you please leave it here for me? I'll be so good this year, I PROMISE!
> Love, Torrie

On Christmas morning, just like every other Christmas before, I woke up extremely early, full of anticipation. Without hesitation, I ran into the living room to see if Santa had come, and there waiting for me, under the multi-colored lit tree, was the doll I had been asking for. This longing was fulfilled, and I was a very happy little girl.

So, maybe you're thinking, *Okay, I can't relate to this. My wants are way deeper than a child's Christmas list.* Or, you might be thinking, *What about the longings that go unanswered?* And I have plenty of moments like those as well. The first memory that comes to mind is when I was eighteen years old, and my grandmother passed away. One day she was dancing across the living room floor, full of life and the sillies, and the next, she was no longer here. Her passing was very unexpected to our family as she had just gone in for a simple routine surgery, and following a few complications, she never woke up. It was devastating. Even though I begged God to intercede, He had a different path, and that meant she wasn't there for all of the major moments in my life. She missed my wedding, the birth of my children, my first garden, canning green beans and salsa, and teaching me how to cook her fried apples (I have tried over and over to get them to taste just like hers since I don't have her recipe). She wasn't there for all of the long talks I needed when I realized what grown-up life was really all about. She was gone, she was unattainable, and this prayer was unfulfilled. Now that is the type of longing I am talking about.

The deepest longing, though, the most agonizing longing, I have ever experi-

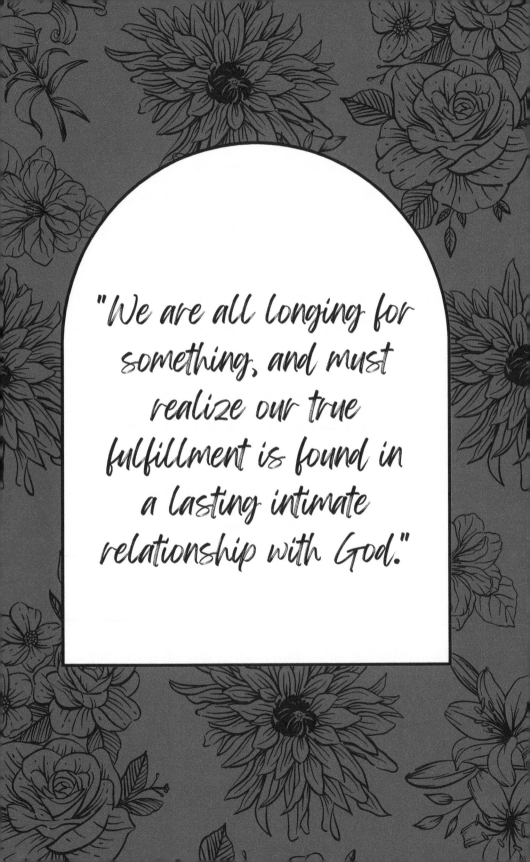

"We are all longing for something, and must realize our true fulfillment is found in a lasting intimate relationship with God."

enced in my life, is the longing for motherhood. The longing to be a mother and not knowing if it would ever happen; looking in the mirror every morning, feeling empty, and wondering if today might be the day I conceive; experiencing the agony of becoming a mother only to lose the baby that once had a little heart beating, fighting to be my child. I've walked this road not once but twice, and, oh, what a devastating place it is. These are the types of things I consider when I speak of longing for something. Those deep hurts that are completely out of our control; the wants that leave us empty; the aches that even a doctor can never fix; the darkest regions in life, where we beg God for a ray of light.

This, my friends, is the LONGING.

What is your deepest longing? Can you recall one yet? Has it captivated your past, present, and future? I hope you relate these stories to your own life, and no matter what you're longing for, you become capable of finding true peace in the arms of Jesus and feel comfort in knowing you are never alone in this battle we call life. We all have struggles, heartbreak, and isolating moments; we are all longing for something and must realize our true fulfillment is found in a lasting intimate relationship with God. I especially hope you see how similar our trials in this modern-day life are to those who lived long ago, which we read about in the Bible, and realize we aren't much different from them. Our hearts and bodies are still created the same, yet our twenty-first-century lives are much faster-paced than theirs were, nevertheless, while waiting for an answer that only God can give, there is no Amazon link to make it arrive any quicker. We are all halted, waiting on His perfect timing and plan. Make the decision today, before turning another page, to open your heart and your mind to the things God wants to teach you during this momentous season, the season of *"LONGING"*.

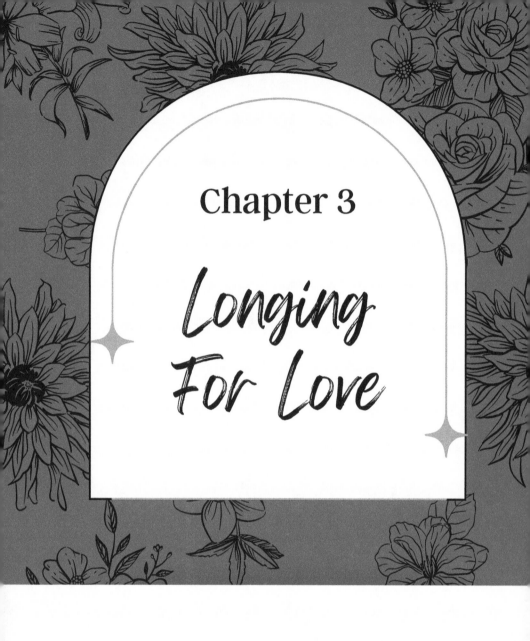

Chapter 3

Longing For Love

Love bears all things,
believes all things, hopes all things,
endures all things. Love never ends...

1 Corinthians 13:7-8a, ESV

Love bears all things, believes all things,
hopes all things, endures all things.
Love never ends...
1 Corinthians 13:7-8a, ESV

I was twelve years old when I started praying for my husband. I prayed every single night for him, not even knowing who he might be. I prayed he would love God, be a good man, and that God would watch over him and guard His life. Growing up as a Southern Baptist pastor's daughter, I was taught I should pray very specifically for my spouse. God knew who he would be, and I wanted my man to be taken care of, so every single night, I prayed for him with intention. When I was fourteen, I attended a youth conference, one that my church had been to every year. At this particular conference, they spoke a lot about waiting for the right one. If you grew up in church, I'm sure you know this type of conference, where they speak a lot about purity and saving yourself for marriage. I had been to youth conferences for a couple of years prior, so I was very familiar with these sorts of purity messages, but one thing I had not heard yet was to "pray specifically." In fact, during this particular sermon, the Pastor instructed us to take out a piece of paper and a pen and write down the exact qualities we desired in our future spouses. Now, this was a twist that spoke directly to my soul. I am somewhat OCD by nature, and I was listening to someone telling me I could write down the distinct details I wanted in my future husband, and that by faith, God was going to deliver him to me in His perfect time. Now, this is the type of task I was most certainly all about! I mean, in 2022 lingo, this would be the same as telling me I am one Amazon click away from obtaining a perfect fiancée. Ummm ... Yes please, and will someone quickly hand this girl a piece of paper!

So without hesitation, I quickly began to write down the most specific details describing the man of my dreams, and I'll give you one guess as to what the starting line was at the top of my paper:

1. TALL, DARK, & HANDSOME ... (of course!)

I wrote the most minute details, down to the type of haircut and shoes he would be wearing. After all, I was going to be a hairstylist and designer one day, so in my fourteen-year-old mindset, this man could not be "uncool" (haha). I'm sure God was just loving the little demands I was quickly jotting down, leaving Him absolutely no room for all of the details HE actually had in mind for my perfect husband. As I reached the end of my paper, I concluded this "little" (quite long) list of things with some swirly handwriting and bubble letters, folded it, and placed it neatly in my Bible. After all, the Bible might as well be a mailbox directly to the heart of God. I figured He would read it often and start working right away on my very perfect man.

So, I will spare you the, unfortunately, long four-year journey of bad experiences and failed relationships until finally meeting my husband, but I do want to share some things that went wrong with this very detailed life plan I had written down that day. After writing out this list, I clung to every word of it. The problem was, I left out some of the most important parts about my future spouse's spiritual relationship with God when I took the sermon quite literally and wrote down the tiniest details about my future husband's appearance. And when I say details, I mean even down to the man must have some "hunky hands." Side note and minor detour right here to explain. My dad had manly hands, and when I was a child, I always noticed little details like this one. It became a joke between my dad and me that whoever I married would have "hunky hands." To help you picture the type: envision manly, willing-to-get-dirty, large, handsome hands. I did not prefer dainty hands or long fingernails on a guy. NO, he must be willing to fix my car or chop some wood (you know, manly, hunky guy stuff). After meeting someone new, I would list all of the little things I liked about them and see what qualities matched my list. During these contemplation scenarios, my Dad would get really serious and say, "Okay, I've got one question for you ... Does he have hunky hands??" When my response was a no or a long pause, he quickly without a doubt would say, "Well then, he's not the one."

Going through life, I dated several tall, dark, and handsome types. I would think of my list and how many checks they marked off of it. The problem with this was, I didn't write about loyalty, honesty, a deeply rooted relationship with God, or things that really mattered for my future. So, every single time I dated someone new, I allowed myself to fully trust the guy because, after all, they had *"most"* of the items on my list marked off. These few relationships ended so painfully, taking significant pieces of my heart and trust with them along the way. I had allowed my longing for a husband and a family to consume my thoughts so much, I didn't seek the correct journey and timing that God had planned for my life. This fault of mine caused me so much heartache, hurt, and pain along the way. I was so clouded by my idea of a written perfect plan, I didn't leave room for God to mold and perfect His own. His plan didn't include my husband at fifteen, sixteen, or seventeen like I thought it would, and if I had just spent those years focusing on God, falling in love with Him, and not thinking that every tall, dark, and handsome guy that crossed my path was the "one," I would have saved myself so much heartbreak and grief.

But seek first the kingdom of God, and His righteousness,
and all these things shall be added to you.
Matthew 6:33, NKJV

I met my husband when I was eighteen. We had a group of mutual friends, and it didn't take long for him to absolutely fall head over heels in love with me, as he begged to take me on a date. (Hahaha, he doesn't like to read either, so the chances of him reading this are slim.) I mean, that's how I remember it, anyways.

I was eighteen, and I had just signed a lease on my very first house. So, that meant there was no more room renting or bumming off of friends for me. I had my own space now, equipped with a fully stocked cooler (I had no fridge), my TV sat on two fabulously stacked crates, where I watched the same three

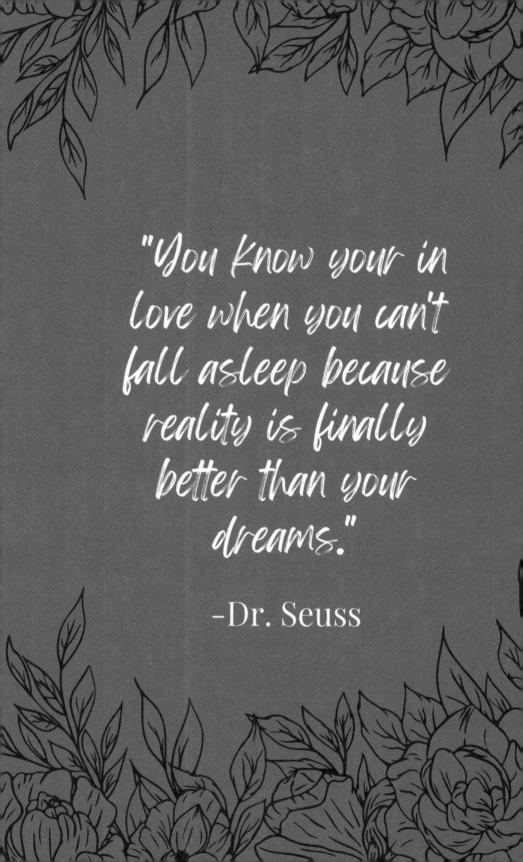

"You know your in love when you can't fall asleep because reality is finally better than your dreams."

-Dr. Seuss

movies on repeat. (After all, who had the money for cable?) I was spending my nights painting walls, making this house my home, and I had fully devoted my life solely to God. For me, this was a completely fresh start after a terrible break-up, and I had entirely committed to living my life only falling more in love with the Lord. This is where I see that God does have a sense of humor because it was literally right after making the plan of self-determination that my phone rang. When I looked down and saw the name "Brenton," my stomach did an unexpected flip. We were friends, but not the type of friends that called each other. When I answered, "Hello?", his response was so romantic (yeah, right) with a loud, "Hey girl!"

We chatted back and forth about my new house and the things we both had going on in our lives at the time. We ended our conversation after a few minutes with him saying I needed to go out with him sometime, and I answered with a very hesitant, "Maybe so."

A few days later, I was at home painting, when I heard an unpredicted knock on the door. Who do you think this surprise visitor might be? Yep, my knight in shining armor, and on a motorcycle, no less. There he was in all of his tall, dark, and handsomeness, asking me to go on a little ride. I was completely reluctant because I was not looking for a relationship at the moment, but I hesitantly agreed as he handed me a helmet, and off we went. As we rode off, I remember how amazing he smelled and holding onto his waist until my knuckles turned white, while also praying to not fall off the back. And it's probably a good thing I was sitting behind him on the darn thing because I'm sure the huge smile on my face ruined the "play-it-cool" vibes I had been working so hard on.

Over the next couple of weeks, this became a normal routine. I would be working at my house, he would drop by, and the short little phone chats turned into hour-long conversations. My cooler disappeared, and he bought me a brand-new fridge (fully stocked, no less). Things were moving super-fast; I was letting myself fall for my friend until I realized what I thought was a big problem: He's. Too. Nice. How is this possible? My radar was going off, and this was just too good to be true. The more I allowed my thoughts to take hold, the more unsure I became about our relationship. I began to pick apart tiny things he was missing from my list. Oh my, but he had some really hunky hands ... but, but, but. Reasons why this wouldn't work flooded my mind, and my worries and fears were getting the best of me. So, on the way home from dinner one night, I randomly blurted out, "I don't know if I can do this!"

"What?" he asked.

"This!" I replied. "All of this! I don't know if I feel the same way about you that you feel about me. I don't know if I'm ready for a relationship like this. I just don't know if all of this is what I want."

The answer he gave to my statement is the moment I fell in love with him. He, without hesitation, replied, "Okay, whatever makes you happy is what I want. If that means you are with someone else, and you are happy, I want that. I don't want to lose you because I know what my feelings are, and if that means I have to wait for you, then I will, but I just want you to be happy."

"STOP!!!!" I shouted. "Stop, right there. I take it back, never mind. I take back every word I just said."

I had never had any man put me before themselves. I had been cheated on and lied to more times than I cared to count, and this genuine guy was sitting there treating me like an absolute queen, AND he put my own happiness before his. This, my friends, was the answer to many prayers, and this was the fulfillment of my longing for a soulmate. He was mine, and I realized this very early on, but I was too scared to admit it because it interrupted how I thought things would happen. The fear I felt, at that moment, of losing him, I knew I never wanted to feel again. He was my missing piece. Brenton didn't check off everything on my list from when I was fourteen, but the list I needed when I was eighteen, nineteen, twenty-five, and even now at thirty-four . . . he still checks it off every single day. I am so thankful God didn't answer some of the prayers I prayed at fourteen. I'm glad He didn't grant the wishes I made during all-night tear fests over the guys I thought were perfect for me. I am so much better off now, with the one God had waiting for me. He is my one true love, and he makes the years of longing for a good man undisputedly worth it.

I share this story because this is where I remember experiencing my first heartbreak; the first real longing experience. Every girl, at some point, has dreamt of having a good man in her life to grow old with, and I'm sure if I asked, you would quickly recall the first love that broke your heart. These encounters create scars on our hearts that last forever and painful memories we can never forget. But, when we endure those difficult seasons of life and allow God to mold us into a more beautiful version of ourselves, our hearts are further prepared for when we actually meet the "right one." Then, we are able to be better spouses, knowing where we have been and having a deeper relationship with God than ever before. I completely believe that if I had met my husband at fourteen, when I really wanted to, we wouldn't be together today. I wasn't ready for him back then because God hadn't completely prepared my heart for our relationship yet. He wasn't ready for me since God was still equipping his life as well (that, and he also had a terrible mustache that would have sent me running for sure, and that's a promise in itself that God always knows best). You can see here how unquestionably more valuable God's timing and precise direction for our life is over our own ideas. God didn't give me a husband exactly when I requested one. He didn't give me the desires of my heart when I begged him to restore my shattered relationship with a cheater. He gave the right one to me after I had endured many broken hearts and in His perfect timing (which was a moment I least expected). Then, when I tried to be in charge again, I thought the man He gave me was too good and ALMOST let him go. Thank the Lord for at least having enough wisdom to retract my words right after speaking them.

Jesus replied,
"You must love the Lord your God with all your heart,
all your soul, and all your mind.
This is the first and greatest commandment."
Matthew 22:37 & 38 NLT

So friend, what are you longing for? What is the desire of your heart? Whatever season of longing you are in right now, He hears you. He is waiting to be the answer to every prayer you are praying. He deeply desires a relationship with us, and He wants us to devote our lives to Him. The truth is, if we pledge our lives to anything other than fully committing to Christ, we will come up short. Since we were created by God and are made in His image, it is impossible for us to be fulfilled without Him as the center of our lives. He is telling us in these two verses from Matthew that loving God with every piece of our existence is the most significant commandment. There is NOTHING more important than falling in love with God and making Him the most important thing in our lives. By loving Him and having complete faith that He will fill the longings of our hearts in the way He has planned, our plans and longings become aligned with His. Then, through Him, we will be satisfied.

Understand, therefore, that the Lord your God is indeed God,
He is the faithful God who keeps His covenant for a thousand
generations and lavishes His unfailing love onto those
who love Him and obey His commands.
Deuteronomy 7:9, NIV

This tells us when we love God as he has commanded us to, He LAVISHES His UNFAILING love onto us. Wow! He asked us to love Him, and in return, He wants to give us a lavish, unfailing type of love. Do you see here how much He loves us? It's unconditional. It's everlasting. It's more fulfilling than any type of love we can find here on earth. When we learn from this love, His lavish unfailing love, then we will understand how to accurately love our spouse and family. Trust Him through the longing and fully devote your life to loving Him like never before.

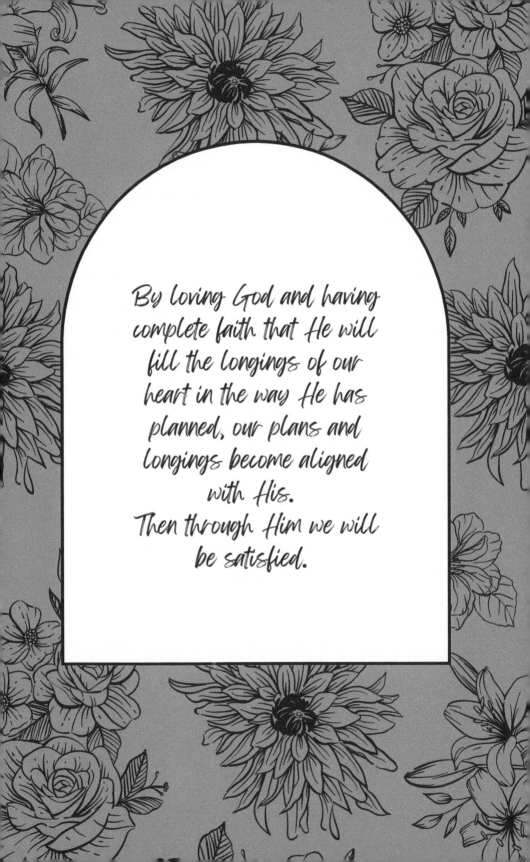

By loving God and having complete faith that He will fill the longings of our heart in the way He has planned, our plans and longings become aligned with His.
Then through Him we will be satisfied.

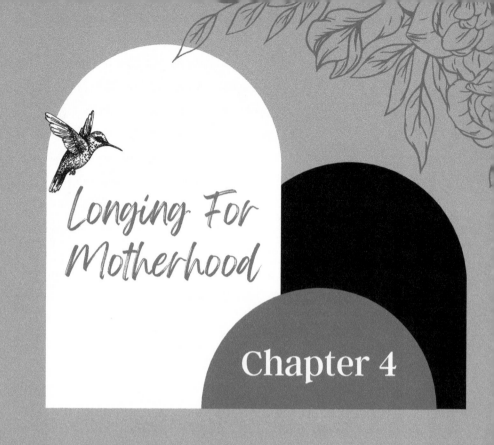

Longing For Motherhood

Chapter 4

Being a mother is
learning about strengths you
didn't know you had...
and dealing with fears you
didn't know existed.
-Linda Wooten

*Being a mother is learning about strengths you didn't know you had...
and dealing with fears you didn't know existed.*
-Linda Wooten, author[4]

On September 29, 2007, we said I do. We had dated for a year and a half, and in most people's minds, that wasn't long enough. For Brenton and I, however, it seemed as though we had been together forever. I knew he was the one I would marry after dating only two weeks. Waiting a year and a half to call this guy my husband, well, it felt like an eternity.

Not long after marriage, we began talking more and more about our goals and dreams of starting a family. We set travel goals and made a checklist of things we wanted to do before we had a baby. We called it our bucket list. We planned exciting adventures in Jamaica (where I was randomly pulled from the crowd and somehow won the resort bootie-shaking contest. Embarrassing. I know. I'm a pretty horrible dancer, so I'm still stumped at how I managed to pull that one off. I basically started convulsing my entire body randomly as fast as I could, and somehow, ya girl won). We went on ski trips, whitewater rafting, flew to NYC, went on hiking adventures, and even skydiving. It was a very busy couple of years, and in our minds, the perfect pre-baby checklist. Once we purchased a new home, which had extra rooms for our future babies, we were immediately ready to fill them. I thought that upon having the "it's time" conversation, I would absolutely be a mother within a few months, max.

So I thought ...

Inevitably, days turned into weeks, and those weeks evolved into months, and I found myself sitting on my porch in mid-March without a baby in my arms. As I held a warm cup of coffee in my hands, I took in the world around me, realizing spring was unavoidably approaching. Even though I didn't want to admit it, I had gone an entire year with an empty womb and no promise of motherhood in my future. Avoiding the chill in the air, I pulled the fluffy blanket tightly around my legs. While gently swaying back and forth on my porch swing, I reflected on each of my friends who had announced their pregnancies over the past few months. This thought stung my heart as I wondered if this would ever be a possibility for us.

For me, my porch was my place of thought. Do you have one of those? The one place where your thoughts come in slightly clearer, and when you're waiting on a word from God, the answer comes in just a little bit louder. Well, this black wooden swing, hand-built by my father-in-law, was my spot. I had spent a lot of time on it during that year, praying and reflecting. I examined my life for flaws while making deals with God to fix the imperfections within it if He would answer my one prayer. Do you do this? Do you ask God for something you deeply long for, and while waiting for that prayer to be answered, you start making deals, negotiations, and promises? Like, "God, if you sell this house, I promise I won't miss a single service at church for six months." Or, "Okay God, if you give us a baby, I promise I will share the news with everyone I meet that You deserve all of the glory and have truly created a miracle child." Does this sound familiar to you? This is the plea of desperation to fill the deep longing you have within. Well, for me, my quiet praying spot had now become the begging swing. In any area of my life where I found a weakness, I traded, negotiated, and begged God. I cleaned out the nooks and crannies of my soul, removed cobwebs in my heart, while begging and pleading to become a mother. Yet, every single month, there was only one line on my pregnancy test. It was the worst feeling. It was the loneliest place. I felt so deeply broken living in this position, stuck in the unknown. I questioned God often. *Would I ever be a mother? Would I have my home full of children just as I had always planned?* I remember talking with friends while going through this waiting period and pouring my crazy heart out to them, only to receive a long blank stare in return. You know it, the kind of stare and look on their face, like they have no idea what you're going through, how to help you, or what to say. Then, they say the one thing that every person who has never been in your pair of

"In spite of the pangs of travail, the longing for motherhood remains the most powerful instinct in woman."

-Joseph Hertz

The Pentateuch and Haftorahs (one-volume edition, 1937

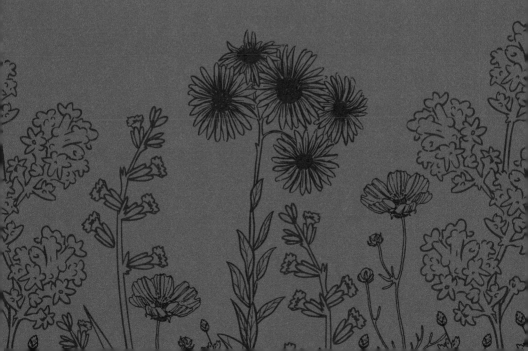

shoes says: "It will happen when you least expect it," or "If you're stressed and think about it too much, it's not going to happen." Now, how is that supposed to help? If I'm expecting to be "expecting" (see what I did there?), how can I think of anything else but that? Or after months of not conceiving, how can I not become a little bit overwhelmed? It's really quite impossible, actually. The truth is, there was nothing anyone could really tell me to make me feel better. I was stuck, with no promise of motherhood in my future, an empty womb, and a weary heart. Have you been in this place? Have you been in this waiting period? Maybe you are there now, and that's why you have picked up this book, or maybe you are in the stage of loss, so you have briefly experienced motherhood, and then every bit of it was ripped away from you. I have been there too, and I will talk more about that in another chapter, but for now, I want you to understand that even in the waiting, GOD IS THERE. He resides in the stillness. He dwells in the unknown. He is even present in the silence. He will never leave us or forsake us. He tells us that in His word.

Fear not, for I am with you;
Be not dismayed, for I am your God;
I will strengthen you, Yes, I will help you,
I will uphold you with my righteous right hand.
Isaiah 41:10, NKJV

Isn't that such a beautiful promise? "Fear not." Those two words alone say abundantly more. "Fear not", meaning, don't be afraid of the unknowns. Do not be fearful of your future, because we are not alone. God is with us, consistently. He will give us the strength to press through the strenuous moments of our journey. He tells us in His word to be not dismayed, for He is our God. Meaning, do not be stressed or worried because we serve the one and only God who is never too busy for us. He is the creator of life and the engineer of everything. I could list, on and on, the magnitudes that God has made, because he is the maker of ALL things.

I know what you're thinking when I say all of those words. Then why? Why, if He is the maker of all of things, the creator of life, and the loving Father to all humankind, why hasn't my one prayer been answered? I cannot answer that question. I can tell you some of the details God showed me during my journey through this place, the place of longing for motherhood.

Answer 1: Benefits of Praying

Though everyone's experience in the journey of motherhood is different, I believe I grew my time of waiting and longing for a child. The prayers and tears I spent on each one of my children made me appreciate how special they truly are. I had to wait on them. I prayed diligently for God's comfort and peace. That waiting and praying placed a higher value on my everyday motherhood journey. Now, please don't paint this perfect picture of me as a patient, kind, soft-spoken, and angelic child-tamer. Because that's unrealistic. The waiting would never be long enough for me to turn into a saint, especially when my two toddlers threw an all-out tantrum in the middle of Starbucks. I think even Mother Teresa would break into a sweat and cut that evil eye during moments like those. However, when days are long and nights are even longer, I remember how blessed I truly am. I reflect on all of the prayers while longing for motherhood, and even on the hardest of hard days, being a mother has more meaning now because of the struggles along the way.

Answer 2: The Importance of Seeing God Speak

Okay. This is one of the most important lessons I learned while waiting for each of my children. You might think, *"Seeing" God Speak? How do you see Him speak? Wouldn't you hear Him?* My answer to those thoughts and questions is this: God speaks to us through his Word, and we can clearly hear Him speaking to us as we read it. The Bible is full of scriptures and life-applicable stories we can relate to and apply to our personal day-to-day life. God uses His scriptures to minister to our significant needs through personal study time, sermons at church, blogs, songs, podcasts, and so many other ways at the most pivotal timing in our lives. The value of God's Word will never depreciate, but when you *"see God speak"*, so directly, so unmistakably right to you, it's a life-changing moment you will never forget, and it creates a personal, intimate relationship with God that lasts forever.

The story that comes to mind when I say "see God speak" is when I first truly experienced it in my own life while I was struggling to conceive. I owned a beauty salon during our "trying" years, and anyone who goes to the salon knows the majority of what goes on there is talking and more talking, or and of course, hair styling. So, everyone who sat in my chair, during this time in my life, pretty much knew we were trying for a baby. In making this announcement, I didn't know there was such a thing as a "waiting period." I thought you just decided to have a baby, and the next month, there was a positive result on the pregnancy test (HA! Boy, was I wrong). So, I had a regular client (in salon lingo, this would be a client who comes in weekly to get her hair styled), and of course, we talked every week about, you guessed it, NOT being pregnant. So, one week, while sitting in my salon chair, she spoke of a visit from a hummingbird. She said she had been praying for something specific and was really struggling in her waiting for an answer from God. She explained her day had been the best in quite some time since God sent a hummingbird that morning as a promise that everything would be okay in the battle she was facing. While hearing her story and watching the glow of excitement beaming from her face, I was completely captivated and knew I had to hear more. So, I asked how this whole scenario came about. She said for as long as she could remember, every time she had a big prayer request, God would send a hummingbird as an affirmation, and shortly after its appearance, things would get better or her prayer would be answered.

Well, after this conversation, I quickly decided I needed a hummingbird too. I prayed on the way home that if God was ever going to give us a child, could He send a hummingbird before me to reassure my soul. Now, if I'm being completely transparent, my faith that this was actually going to happen wasn't very strong. I would even say I was probably testing God at this point, because in my mind, I was already supposed to be a mother, and I was utterly desperate for any fragment of a sign it was a possibility. However, I prayed and kept my eyes wide open for my hummingbird. Now, I know you're probably just dying to know what happened next, and it really might blow your mind, because

Even in the waiting,
GOD IS THERE.
He resides in the
stillness.
He dwells in the
unknown.
He is even present
in the silence.
He will never leave
us or forsake us.

mine was quite blown myself.

The following Sunday when we arrived home from church, I was greeted by a very exhausted hummingbird that had somehow been trapped in my garage. Yes, in my garage! It was anxiously flying back and forth, from one side of the garage to the next. It kept landing on our garage track and resting for a few seconds before flying to the other side, so you could tell it had been at this for a while. Well, what a darn blessing this was, I thought. I prayed for a hummingbird, and wouldn't you know it, I was going to have one die right here in my house. I was a bit panicked, not knowing how to get this thing out before it really cursed my life forever, and I never became a mother. My first thought was to persuade it out the garage door to freedom, however, I quickly realized this was absolutely not going to end well. So, after chasing it with a broom for a few minutes, I decided it was time for a new plan. I slowly climbed on the top of a tall ladder and simply stood there with my finger in the air, while continuously praying for a miracle. I don't know why I thought this would work, after all, my Nanny told me the story of a time she tried to catch a hummingbird, and before she could even let it go, it had pecked her hand about a hundred times. Nevertheless, here I was. So, as I stood there on the ladder looking as tree-ish as possible, it started to come near me. It got closer and closer until, suddenly, I felt tiny little feet lightly perched on my finger. I stayed so still and tried to gather my panicking thoughts, while slowly reaching my other hand up to grab it. Surprisingly, it never moved! It stayed so still and calm as I carried it down the ladder and out of the garage to safety. This tiny little bird looked me in the eyes and calmly watched as I opened my hands. It stood, still perched in my palm as if it were peering into my very soul. At that moment, I felt it was thanking me, and I knew in my heart, God sent this little hummingbird to me as a promise.

That was the big moment I "saw" God speak to me. I saw Him answer the small prayer I had prayed. It was almost so crazy, no one else would under-stand the importance of it, but I knew exactly what this meant and how im-pactful it was to my future. At that moment, I knew I would be a mother. I knew this longing would be fulfilled in His perfect timing. I realized it wasn't me that was the problem. God didn't want my trades and sacrifices in order to supply me with the promise of motherhood, because he had already paid all of my debts on the cross long ago. Telling this story floods my heart with so many emotions because this one thing changed me forever. It completely changed the way I viewed God and His astounding love for us. God has used hummingbirds in my life from that day forward.

So, my dear friend, in your longing journey, ask Him for confirmation. Invite Him to reveal His direction for your journey. He will show up. He wants to speak to us. These moments may make the pain of your longing sting a little less. Seeing God "speak" to us is so important to strengthen our faith, and it was through this journey, I learned how important an undeniable faith in God really is.

Chapter 5

Unforeseen News

For I know the plans I have for you,
declares the Lord, plans for welfare
and not for evil, to give you
a future and a hope.

Jeremiah 29:11, ESV

For I know the plans I have for you, declares
the Lord, plans for welfare and not for evil,
to give you a future and a hope.
Jeremiah 29:11, ESV

Anyone who has been trying to conceive a baby for a few months without becoming pregnant has probably already taken a few negative pregnancy tests, or if you're like me, a lot of them. Aren't they just daunting? Month after month, test after test, and negative after negative. Nothing ruins a day any quicker than thinking you are pregnant, only to find out that you are not. That crushing moment reminds you of the month ahead repeating the same process all over again, charting ovulation, trying again, and waiting to find out if it worked. In the season of "trying for a baby," it feels as if every single month creeps along like a year, and a year might as well be an eternity. You build up hope of becoming pregnant time and time again only to see another negative staring back at you. It's crushing.

At this point in my fertility journey, it had been a few months since we started trying for our first baby, and I was already a stressed-out mess. I am a planner by nature, and some might say a bit OCD about controlling all of the areas in my life ... I like to handle all of the things and fix all of the problems, and I LOVE a good three to five-year plan. I've never been great at handing over responsibility to someone else. And oh dear Jesus, take the wheel if I have to wait on something to get done in the way I think it should. So, you can imagine my surprise at not being a "mother" already after a few months of trying to conceive. My heart was ready for motherhood, and my mind was convincing me it wasn't going to happen. I began to ask myself things like: *Is something wrong with me? Will I ever be able to conceive?* I was scared and constantly worrying myself to death that my plan of having four children might never be-

It is essential to acquire endurance from the little battles we face today, to better prepare our hearts and minds for the bigger battles we will encounter in the future.

come a reality. After much thought, I decided I would make an appointment with my OB-GYN to see what kind of advice she could give me. At this point, it had only been a few months since we began trying to conceive, but as I said before, I had a plan, and I was already months behind.

On the day of my appointment, I sat on the table, waiting for my doctor to come into the exam room. I anticipated she would have a professional answer for me, and I had complete faith she would tell me what I was doing wrong and how to become pregnant with a baby in the next month. As I sat nervously on the table fidgeting with the sheet they call a robe, I heard a little tap on the door, and the doctor walked in. Before she even had time to get settled in her tiny stool, I quickly began blubbering all of the thoughts that had been whirling around in my head. I explained I thought I had charted correctly, hit ovulation dates, taken my prenatal vitamins, and many other things, and I thought it all might help the process, yet nothing had worked, and I still wasn't pregnant. After I was all done stating my case, I sat quietly so she could tell me the magical solution to my problem. She looked at me with unfazed eyes and told me all of the "by the book" reasons why this was completely normal. She explained I should stop thinking about wanting a baby so badly because stress is a deterrent to getting pregnant for some women. And then, she hit me with the one I was least prepared for of all: "We are not concerned until you hit the one-year mark of infertility." *Ummm, say what now, sister?? You are going to do nothing for an entire year?* I mean, I have been trying for a few months, and it already feels like an eternity. How was I supposed to waste a year of my life waiting to become a mother?

There were so many things I wanted to tell her. Instead, I tightly pressed my lips together, forced a smile, and fought back the tears trying to engulf my eyes. I will never forget that day as I left the office feeling completely helpless. Knowing how far I was from help made me feel like I had just been punched in the gut. It felt as if I would never become a mother, and the year that lay before me might as well have been a decade in my mind.

After that doctor's appointment, I was an absolute wreck, and I knew there was only One that could help me now. That was Jesus. Isn't it interesting how sometimes Jesus is our last resort? Isn't it a bit backward? We serve a proven miracle worker, but we don't fully place our problems in His hands until there are no other hands to place them in. Oh, that stings just typing it. You might be thinking, *I always pray and ask God first, and I have been begging God for a miracle. But, here I am still waiting, unfulfilled, and empty.* And, trust me, I have been there. I have been in that spot, living life, begging God for a miracle, and fully trusting He could deliver it, continually waiting day after day. But, friend, here is the difference. You can place your prayers in God's hands today, but until you stop picking them back up tomorrow, you will never be free from them. Until you fully allow Him to handle it and do the work in his perfect timing, you will never find peace. Peace doesn't dwell in the fulfillment of the prayer you are asking for. Peace rests in trusting God's timing is right and knowing he has a perfect plan for your life.

> *I have said these things to you, that in me you may*
> *have peace. In the world you will have tribulation.*
> *But take heart; I have overcome the world.*
> John 16:33, ESV

This scripture reminds us we will have trials in the world and in our daily lives, but nothing is too hard for God. He wants us to know He has already overcome the world and every obstacle that resides in it. No matter how worked up you get, how bothered, and how busy you stay, it doesn't accelerate God's perfect timing. So, find rest today in knowing that when it's right, it will be. And when His plan is not your own, it will be okay.

When we hit our one-year mark, I went back to the doctor. This time, she began the next process of our infertility journey, which was to start running tests to see if everything was working properly for both of us. This part of the journey unavoidably involved Brenton and landed him in a very awkward doctor's office visit. If you've been down this road, then I'm sure you know what I am referring to.

Peace doesn't dwell in the
fulfillment of the prayer you
are asking for. Peace rests in
trusting that God's timing is
just right and knowing he has
a perfect plan for your life.

Not only that, but we rejoice in our sufferings, knowing that suffering produces endurance, and endurance produces character, and character produces hope, and hope does not put us to shame, because God's love has been poured into our hearts through the Holy Spirit who has been given to us.

Romans 5:3–5, ESV

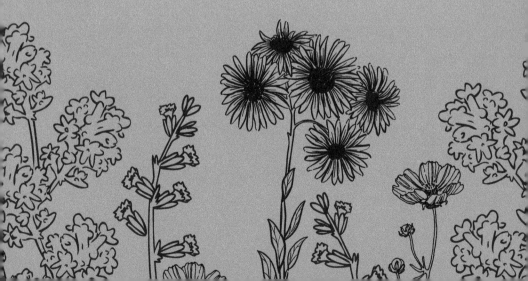

Late on a Thursday night, I was on my way home from work when Brenton called with the news we had been waiting for—the results from his testing that changed our lives forever. I listened intently to every word as he told me the details. He explained, "The semen counts were low, shapes were damaged, and the speeds were slower than needed for conception to take place." The doctor believed this was a result of a previous injury to Brenton when he was electrocuted on a powerline. It was, indeed, a miracle that he survived, and he went through a very extensive recovery process. At the time of the accident, they told him he would likely suffer from some side effects in the future due to his injuries and burns. But, no one mentioned the possibility of sterilization or damage in that particular area, until now. We were both in complete shock, and this was news we were not expecting. For a year, I had considered all possibilities that could have been hindering my body from conceiving, but the thought never crossed my mind that it could be his. Helplessness flooded my soul. In my mind, the possibility of motherhood was slipping away, and there was nothing I could do about it.

Not only that, but we rejoice in our sufferings, knowing that suffering produces endurance, and endurance produces character, and character produces hope, and hope does not put us to shame, because God's love has been poured into our hearts through the Holy Spirit who has been given to us.
Romans 5:3-5, ESV

With each passing day, I became more empty than ever. I prayed many surrendering prayers; I made deals with God, set deadlines, and tried to walk the straightest line I could. In my heart, I knew I was doing everything possible to be worthy of motherhood. Yet, at the end of every single month, my womb remained empty. Thinking back to this time, I wish I could go back and talk to that version of myself. If I could, this is what I would say: You are worthy, just the way you are. You are perfectly made, without even trying to be perfect. You are called for a purpose; there is significance to this journey, and you are already a "mother," because the heart you have right now unconditionally loves those babies you will have one day. The purpose of this suffering is to produce a specific quality in you that could not be obtained without this journey. God loves you for you. The tired you, the sad feelings, the broken parts, the imperfect version, he loves all of you to the deepest core. Therefore, nothing you will do can make you more worthy of motherhood or God's love because you are ... WORTHY. Today is just not your time. Today is what is not perfect, and tomorrow might not be either, and that's okay. Because, one day in the future, the timing will be right. God's time.

My dear friend, I want you to read over those words as if I am talking straight to you. If you are going through this type of hard season, I want you to know that God unconditionally loves you, and He has a plan for your life. The difficult trials you are going through today might not make sense for many years to come, but one day, you might understand and be able to use your difficult story for His good. As the scripture in Romans tells us, suffering produces endurance, character, and hope. Without suffering, how can we obtain those things? It's essential to acquire endurance from the little battles we face today, to better prepare our hearts and minds for the bigger battles we will encounter in the future. Embrace the difficult journey and allow Him to produce enduring character within our lives. Find hope in realizing God has already shown us His unconditional love by sending Christ to die for us while we were sinners. He sees us as worthy, He calls us His children, and He is the creator of unconditional love. Today, I pray you to find peace in knowing that you are worthy of God's love in whatever season of life you are in.

When we were utterly helpless, Christ came at just the right time and died for us sinners. Now, most people would not be willing to die for an upright person, though someone might perhaps be willing to die for a person who is especially good. But God showed us His great love for us by sending Christ to die for us while we were still sinners.
Romans 5:6-8, NLT

Chapter 6

God's Promise

"I will bless her, and moreover, I will give you a son by her. I will bless her and she shall become nations; kings of peoples shall come from her."
God said, "No, but Sarah your wife shall bear you a son, and you shall call his name Isaac. I will establish my covenant with him as an everlasting covenant for his offspring after him."

Genesis 17:16 & 19, ESV

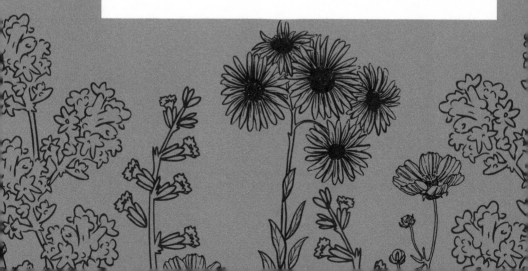

*"I will bless her, and moreover, I will give you a son by her. I will bless
her, and she shall become nations; kings of peoples shall come from her."
God said, "No, but Sarah your wife shall bear you a son, and you shall
call his name Isaac. I will establish my covenant with him as
an everlasting covenant for his offspring after him."*
Genesis 17:16 & 19, ESV

I will never forget the first time this scripture came to me. It was so clear and evident God was telling me I was meant to be a mother. Some might say this scripture was meant for Sarah and Sarah alone. But God gave us His Word to speak to us. He gave us scripture to guide our lives, and God used this story of Abraham and Sarah to impact my life in a way I will never get over.

If you don't know anything about Abraham and Sarah, let me be the first to tell you about one of God's many miracles before I tell you how God used this story in my life. Abraham was one of God's chosen people. Prior to this scripture in Genesis 17, God promised land to Abraham and to his son. Abraham replied to God that he had no son and wondered how this would come to be. God replied to Abraham, He would indeed give him a son, and on top of that, an entire nation. If we fast forward years down the road, Abraham was now ninety-nine years old and his wife, Sarah, was ninety. God spoke to Abraham again saying He would bless them with a son and that his name would be Isaac. Not only did He promise a son, but He promised a multitude of people, princes, and kings from his lineage, as long as Abraham kept God's covenants. Now, when Abraham and Sarah heard this news, they laughed. They questioned God with a chuckle, saying, "I am ninety-nine, and she is ninety? How on earth would we have a baby now after all of these years of not being able to become pregnant?" God's response can be summed up as: I'm about to show you, because this time, next year, you will be holding him in your arms, and you will name him Isaac. Sure enough, the Bible tells us Isaac is born and blessed from that day forward. His children and his children's children reaped the blessings, and they were given all God had promised to them.

Okay, now that we are all caught up on the story, let me share how God used it in my life. At the end of March, on a regular Sunday morning, I was getting ready for church, thinking about the week ahead. I considered where I was in my cycle, when it would be a good time to take a pregnancy test, and when I would be considered late for my period. It was all in the upcoming week, and this was the time I looked forward to every single month. If you've been here, you know the drill. Week one and two, try try try... Week three, the countdown, constant thoughts of, "Did one and two work?" And then, in week four, start taking pregnancy tests, and pray, pray, pray for a positive result. So, there we were, leading up to week four and also just passing our one-year mark of trying to conceive. It was an all-around emotional place to be in.

During the church service that day, as the pastor opened his Bible, I glanced at the screen to see where he would be reading from. *Genesis 17: 16 & 17* were typed out in bold text. As he began to read the verses, I felt the presence of God surrounding me, and it was as if He Himself was speaking these words directly to me.

I will bless her, and moreover, I will give you a son by her. I will bless her, and she shall become nations; kings of peoples shall come from her." Then Abraham fell on his face and laughed and said to himself, "Shall a child be born to a man who is a hundred years old? Shall Sarah, who is ninety years old, bear a child?"
Genesis 17:16-18, ESV

The sermon he preached that day was titled, "God's Promises." During this sermon, he spoke of the promise God made to Abraham and Sarah on that day, as we read in Genesis 17. This promise was so much more than a promise of a son to them. It was also the promise of blessings upon that son's children and their children to come. It was a promise to mend Sarah's broken heart that so deeply longed for a child for most of her lifetime. It was the promise of a blessing that was seven times what she requested and prayed for. Wow! Can we let that just sink in for a minute, friend? I mean, that's some impeccable timing, and this shows us that the waiting period in Sarah's life was significant. Upon hearing this news, the biggest change took place in my heart as I ugly cried the majority of the service, realizing the importance of God's plan over mine for my life. The moment his sermon was over, I practically ran to the altar to place all of my worries at Jesus' feet, and as I was there at the altar, God promised to me a son. At that moment, as I cried out to God, I knew in my heart I was going to be a mother. Typing this today fills me with so much emotion, and my eyes are filled with tears as I recall the lasting significance this one single moment made on my entire life.

I remember just how defeated I felt walking in the door of church that day and then, how full of life I was walking out, with the promise of motherhood God had given to me. It was so much more than just a promise. It was a break in the silence. It was a link that had been missing during my waiting period. Do you know what I mean there? I had felt so isolated from God in the months prior. I was continually asking for a prayer to be answered, and every month, it was going unfulfilled. As I prayed to God for answers to the many questions I had, I felt silence in return. It was as if He wasn't hearing me at all. Oh, but He was, and He hears you too. He is just whispering to you, in His perfect timing. When your time is right, my daughter, I will show you the perfect plan I have for your life. For some, this could mean conceiving a baby of your own, or for others, this might mean adopting a child who longs for parents with that same deep anticipation as you hold in your heart for motherhood. Whatever your specific journey is, God will reveal it to you.

Let's think for a moment how different things may have been if Sarah had become a mother when she first asked God to fulfill that longing in her life. How many things may have changed if a child had been given in her timing instead of God? The first thought that comes to mind is the name of her son, Isaac, would be different. Verse 17 says, "Abraham laughed" when God told him that he and Sarah would have a son. He laughed at God! It says he fell on his face and laughed, so it sounds like he thought that was pretty hilarious.

Find peace in knowing that everything which takes place in your "today" considerably affects the results of your "tomorrow".

Then, in the next chapter, when Sarah was told she would have a son at ninety, guess what she did? Yes, she laughed too. God even called her out on it saying, "Do you think this is too hard for me?" Of course, they stopped laughing at that point, and I absolutely know I would have too. Later in the Bible, Isaac had a son named Jacob, whose name was later changed to Israel, and pretty much everyone born in the world thereafter came from his lineage. Hence, the phrase, "the children of Israel." If you follow this lineage of Abraham and his son Isaac, and the children of Isaac and so on, eventually, down the line, you will arrive at Jesus' birth. *What? Jesus is a distant relative to Isaac?* This blew my mind when I read it. Are you seeing the effects of God's plan yet? The significance of Jesus' birth is literally the most important birth of all time as He is the Promised Savior of all men, the Messiah, Son of God, and Prince Of Peace. I could continue all day listing the magnificent names of our Lord, but the purpose here is for you to see how many details might have been affected if ONE plan wasn't done as God instructed it to be. How much of this lineage do you think might have changed if Isaac wasn't the long-awaited promised son of Abraham and Sarah? I can tell you my thoughts, and it's that this one tiny part in the story would have immensely changed the outcome of everything because there is so much purpose behind every intricate detail that God orchestrates. As we realize these truths, I'm eternally thankful to God that His plan was more essential than anything Sarah could have ever imagined. Now that we see how timing changes everything, we can also see God's timing is greater and more important than anything we could ever design or plan for our own lives. So, I want you to ask yourself these questions: How does this make you view where you are in your life today? Do you feel like God has a significant purpose for the obstacles you have encountered along your journey? And can you see He is strategically working behind the scenes to create the most perfect destination for your future?

Dear friend, I am sending you air hugs today for comfort, and I want you to find peace in knowing everything which takes place in your "today" considerably affects the results of your "tomorrow." So embrace the waiting, hard days, results that make no sense, traffic delays, burnt dinners, stubbed toes, and negative tests, because each of these unseemingly significant things that you assume were meant to harm you, God actually sent them for the good of your future.

Chapter 7

Caught By Surprise

The Lord said, "I will surely return to you about this time next year, and Sarah your wife shall have a son." And Sarah was listening at the tent door behind him.

Genesis 18:10, ESV

The Lord said, "I will surely return to you about this time next year, and Sarah your wife shall have a son." And Sarah was listening at the tent door behind him.
Genesis 18:10, ESV

The sun shone so brightly through my bedroom window, and like every other morning, it was telling me it was time to get out of bed. I preferred this method of waking up by the sun over an alarm clock blaring its ridiculous loud beeps any day of the week, and this particular morning, I quickly opened my eyes with a big debate in my mind. This was the Thursday following the significant "Promise" sermon, which also happened to the Thursday when I was five days late for my menstrual cycle. I must note, I had already been taking pregnancy tests pretty much every day of the week that I was late. You see, I had once been twelve days past my projected start date before, and those were some really emotional weeks when I just kept thinking I was pregnant only to be greeted with nature's monthly gift almost two weeks late. But, this week felt different from all of the weeks prior, because I had a promise from God, and I was really trying to completely trust Him and remember that His timing and plan are perfect.

My normal morning routine started with rolling out of bed and shuffling my feet into the bathroom to brush my teeth. That morning, as I stood there looking in the mirror, vigorously brushing my teeth, I caught a glimpse of a clear gallon-sized baggie hanging out of the basket in my toilet room. It was the bag of lab pregnancy tests my friend had given me when she no longer needed to take tests anymore. I thought I had taken all of them, but seeing the bag hanging there made me curious. I finished brushing my teeth and went over to see if there were any left. Now, I probably should have avoided this temptation, because every woman knows if there was a test left in this bag, and I was five days late, I would definitely be peeing on it. But, this time, I was torn because Brenton and I had already decided if I hadn't started by Saturday morning, I would take a test with him there. I picked up the bag and the last little white packet dropped to the bottom. There was one left. *Ehhhh*, ya' girl was really torn. However, I dropped the bag back into the basket and made my way into the kitchen. I walked to the refrigerator and quickly opened the door as if something inside held the answer to my dilemma. I stood there, staring up and down, supposedly looking for something to eat for breakfast, but the only thing I could see were pregnancy tests. That is literally all that consumed my mind.

So, what do you think happened at that moment? Did I run out the door, get in my car, and out of the house, so I would keep my word to my husband and, by faith, wait until Saturday? OR, did I close the refrigerator, turn around, quickly walk straight into the bathroom, and take that dang test? Yup, that's me, your impatient nosey friend, who couldn't take it and caved under the pressure. I sat and prayed for two lines. I knew God's promise; I knew He had spoken to me that very week, and I knew I was truly meant to be a mother. The one thing I just didn't know yet was when God was going to deliver that promise. So, I sat there watching and waiting. As the line became clearer, my heart was beating rapidly with anticipation of what the result would be ...

ONE LINE. That's all. AGAIN. Another negative. I exhaled a big breath and closed my eyes to help contain the flood of emotions that were trying to take hold of me. I held back tears as I reminded myself of what made this time different from all of the rest, and it was the promise I now held in my heart. The specific promise from God was something I never had before. This test did not mark the end of my journey. It just meant that day was not my time for motherhood. I held tightly to the thought that the next month might be.

I prayed a lot over the next two days. I knew I still had to take a test with Brenton because that's what we had said we would do together. He had been excited about it this time, so I didn't want to crush him with the news I already knew.

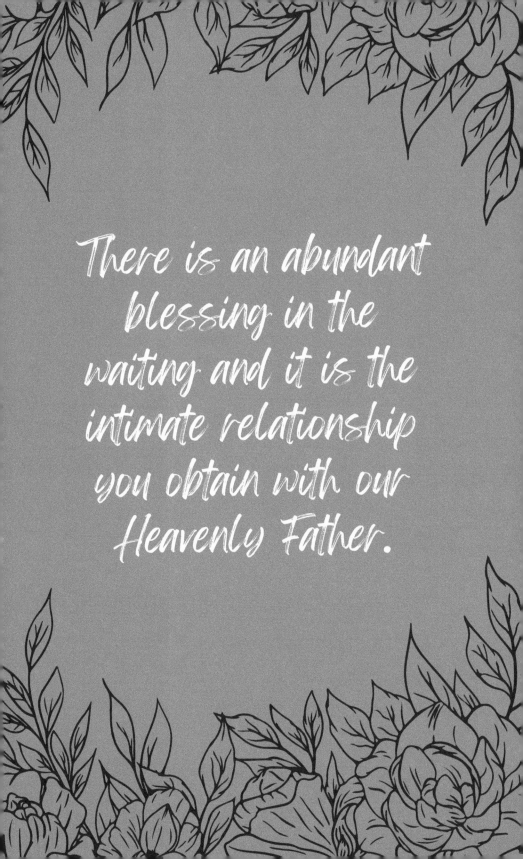

There is an abundant blessing in the waiting and it is the intimate relationship you obtain with our Heavenly Father.

We used to have a "date day" one Saturday each month. Date days have always been one of my absolute favorite traditions. We have never been a couple to like date *nights* because we typically go to bed early; call us old souls or just plain lame, if you will. I don't mind. I'll take either one. Our date day would typically consist of hitting a trendy coffee shop, browsing the aisles at Target, and getting lunch somewhere a bit out of the ordinary.

On this particular "Date Day," we had a test to take before we got ready to go out. Brenton asked if I had picked up the "test" for our "Big Testing Day" (insert his goofy face and animated eyebrow raises while waving his hands around in the air). I nonchalantly laughed and answered, "Yes, and I'm going to take it now" (As if I didn't already take one in my moment of weakness on Thursday). So, I grabbed the box of digital tests I had purchased at Walgreens the day before and headed into the bathroom for yet another negative test.

I laid the test on the bathroom counter and started vigorously brushing my teeth, trying to ignore the ticking time clock blinking on the little digital screen. After I brushed for what felt like ten minutes, I banged the water out of my toothbrush and returned it back to my brush holder. I closed my eyes for a second and opened them again, glancing down. It was still loading! Oh, my gracious; I thought this was a better idea than watching the watermark climb to the top of the test on the traditional type of test, but this was taking forever. I was about to turn into a crazy person and bust this test open to see what the little strip looked like on the inside rather than waiting for this ridiculous clock that had been whirling around forever. As I stood there, staring into the mirror, thoughts swirling like a cyclone in my mind, I heard Brenton's voice yell, "BABE, what does it say?" A bit startled, I closed my eyes and glanced down at the test one more time. Words were now in view on the tiny screen ... I blinked as I read the word PREGNANT in bold letters. I could not believe it! And when I say I could not believe it, I genuinely could not. Tears were streaming down my face as I tried to wrap my mind around the meaning of the first positive test I had ever received.

I forced my feet to move from their frozen position on the bathroom floor. As soon as I walked around the corner into my bedroom, Brenton saw the look on my face and said, "NO WAY???"

I said, "Yes, well, I think so. It says pregnant!" We were in complete shock as we embraced each other and immediately decided I should chug a bottle of water and take another test to be 100% sure. After all, this would be a miracle baby, because on paper, just a few weeks prior, it wasn't medically possible. As the result came into view on the next test, the words still read the same. I was indeed pregnant! I was really going to be a mother. All I could do was cry as those words sank into my mind for the rest of the day. I was holding a little life within me. I was chosen and officially someone's mommy.

I still have a hard time wrapping my thoughts around God's impeccable timing. I have experienced His promises and the fulfillment of His promises. But, it still blows my mind every time I recall them. But, that's how God is, mind-blowing! It took a year to become pregnant, but God was there with me, sending little hummingbirds every single week, while I prayed for Him to show His presence to me. And just when I was ready to give up, and had scientific proof my dreams were no longer possible, He sent a significant message promising me a son. Only God can do that, and it is so important to acknowledge Him. There is an abundant blessing in the waiting and it is the intimate relationship you obtain with our Heavenly Father.

I have talked with a lot of women, and when I tell them the stories of God's faithfulness in my life, they are amazed, but they don't believe God could speak to them in such a way. My question to that statement is this: Have you let Him? Have you really listened to see if He has spoken to you? Have you looked up from your phone to see the hummingbird in your path? God is wanting to draw close to you during your waiting, suffering, and struggles, but we have to be willing to notice Him. We must have complete faith He is there and open our eyes to visualize what He is telling us.

Therefore, the Lord longs to be gracious to you; And therefore,
He waits on high to have compassion on you. For the Lord is a

"The same longing desire we endure for the aspirations of our heart, God experiences this desire over us."

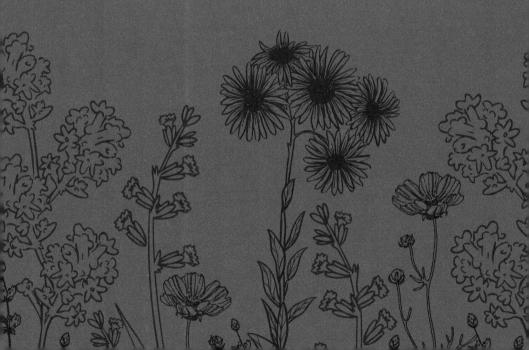

God of justice; Blessed are all those who long for Him.
Isaiah 30:18, NASB

This scripture tells us the Lord longs for us. Did you get that? He truly deeply longs for us! He longs to be gracious and patiently waits to have an intimate relationship with us. This is eye-opening. This verse tells us the same longing desire we endure for the aspirations of our heart, God experiences this same desire over us. Wow! He desperately has compassion for His children; Don't make Him wait for you. Listen to the whispers of His magnificent voice and lean into His gracious embrace. He is there waiting.

Here's my prayer for you, my dear friend.

I pray whatever you long for today, you completely lay it down at Jesus' feet. I pray your deepest dreams are answered and that one thing you lay in bed at night crying for, is appointed in the way God has planned for your life. I pray your soul is drawn closer than ever to the Lord, and your eyes are opened to the little messages God sends you in your everyday routines. I hope you feel his comforting nudges in every vital way He sends them and you receive a strength you never knew possible when your last bit of hope runs out.

AMEN.

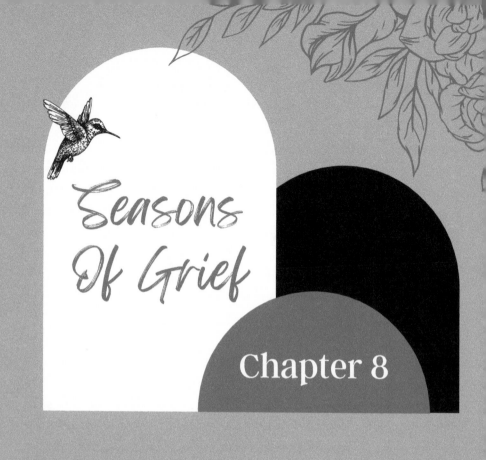

Seasons Of Grief

Chapter 8

The Lord is near to the
brokenhearted and
saves the crushed in spirit.

Psalm 34:18, ESV.

The Lord is near to the brokenhearted and
saves the crushed in spirit.
Psalm 34:18, ESV

It had been six years since I received my first positive pregnancy test. During this time, I experienced the wondrous joys of motherhood, as I became a mother of a handsome little boy, and not long after, an energetic little girl. It was through these years, I was able to fully embrace everything motherhood had to offer. It was a beautiful season of living in God's promise, spiritual growth, and many changes as I matured as a person, Christian, and mother. In March 2017, we finished building our forever home. Our farmhouse. This was a goal we had dreamt of for a long time. We had sketched out many possibilities: building a farmhouse, starting a farm, and owning a business constructing the dreams of others through designing, building, and remodeling homes. This was the year we became Willowbrook.

Those of you that have known us for a while might know us by Willowbrook Builders or Willowbrook Farm. Maybe you have come into our coffee shop, *Willowbrook Grounds*, or maybe you have followed our journey from the beginning when I published my first blog on the Willowbrook Farm Life website. In all of our endeavors, Willowbrook became our face for everything.

When we moved into our newly built home, I wasted no time before planting willows by the brook. Our land had the most peaceful, winding little creek, and right next to it, I envisioned these willow trees growing tall with long limber branches swaying in the wind, back and forth, this way and that, marking the start of this new adventure. We planned to measure our growth by the height of the trees, and just like the peace I felt when I watched them blowing in the wind, so would the presence of God's peace be on this farm. With every plan set in place, a few being smoothly marked off the list, I felt the next season of our lives would be the most perfect yet. My, oh my, how our ideas of perfection are not the plans of God.

Soon, after we got settled into our new home, people began to ask when we would have another child. We had two beautiful children, and the plan was still the same for having two more. Everyone thought that was the craziest idea, having more than two children. They murmured things like, "You have the perfect number already, and one of each, a boy first and then a girl. Why do you need more?"

I ignored their remarks every single time and quickly responded by saying, "We built our home to accommodate four kids, and those empty rooms will be filled." Little did they know, for three years, we had never really prevented pregnancy after our daughter. We knew the struggles we had to conceive both of them. So, there we were with our son, Bentley Mac (five), our daughter, Baize Willow (three), and the hopeful prayer of having another baby in this farmhouse we had worked so hard to build.

I am longing for your deliverance, LORD, and
Your instruction is my joy.
Psalm 119:174, ESV

On July 4th, in our usual "running behind" fashion, we were getting ready to go to a friend's house for a 4th of July celebration. As I rushed around, getting things together for the cookout, I remembered I was a few days late for my menstrual cycle. I stood motionless over the farm sink, now distracted from the to-do list laying on the counter, and my eyes were fixed in a daze staring out the kitchen window. As I stood there debating whether to take a pregnancy test now or wait until the morning, a little hummingbird suddenly appeared and began fluttering around my window. Considering this was one of the communication pieces between me and God, I took this as a sign from Him, and if you know me at all by this point, I'll give you one second to guess which option I chose.

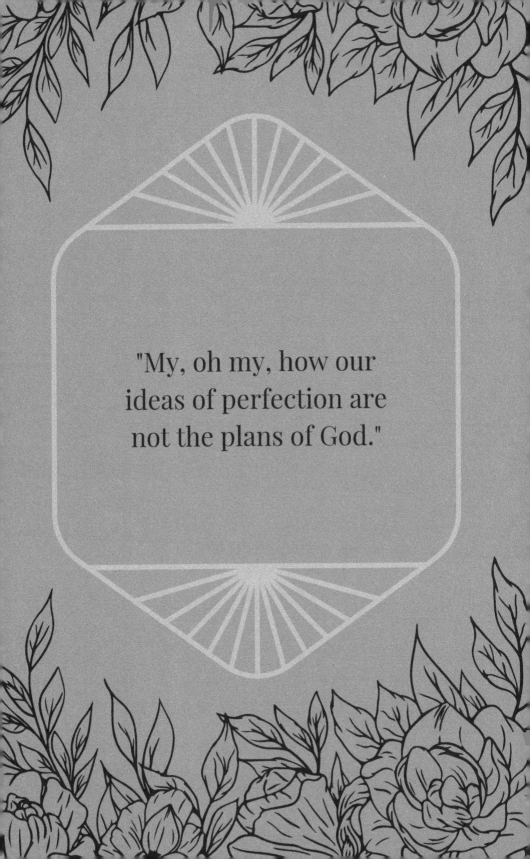

"My, oh my, how our ideas of perfection are not the plans of God."

Pause.

Yes! I sprinted to the bathroom and grabbed my bulky bag of pregnancy tests. By this point, I was a professional at test-taking and purchasing. I had tried all of the brands, from the most expensive to the least, and found the cheap one works just as well as the overpriced two-pack at the retail store (especially when you've taken more negative than not. Why spend so much money?).

I figured how many days late I was and exactly how many weeks pregnant I would be if the test was positive, as I sat waiting for the line to become visible. (Now would be a good time to enter some Jeopardy music as we wait. Shall I sing for you?) After a few minutes, I lifted the test up to the light to make it a bit more clear what I thought I was seeing. There was a tiny pink tint of a line. A very faint positive. My heart was doing this strange sort of speed up with excitement and then sinking with panic rotation over and over, as multiple scenarios ran through my mind. I added up the days, and at this point, I would have been almost five weeks pregnant. I thought back to the positive test for my daughter Baize that I had taken at a little over three weeks pregnant, and it was obviously two dark pink lines. I didn't know what this meant, but I knew the pit in my stomach was making me feel very uncomfortable.

Over the next week and a half, I took test after test, and each day anxiously watched as the line grew darker, little by little. Every time I took a pregnancy test and witnessed the slightest bit of change, my hope grew that everything would be okay with our unborn baby. I was held captive by the unknown until I was far enough along to have my first ultrasound.

On Sunday morning, the week of our appointment, we entered the church doors with our little ones holding our hands. We hugged and greeted our friends, making small talk on the way to our pew, and scooted into our seats, just as service was beginning. I could sense Brenton's fixed gaze on me as if I was a ticking time bomb that just might explode at any moment, and as he reached for my hand, I held it tight. Our pastor walked onto the stage, greeted everyone with a few jokes just as he normally does, and then opened the service by announcing our youth pastor would be delivering the sermon. I was excited about this. I enjoyed hearing our youth pastor preach because he always had relatable stories he enjoyed telling, and his light-hearted preaching style was just what I needed to start my week on a positive note. He came onto the stage, cracked a few jokes, and then he gathered a more serious face and told us to turn in our Bibles to Genesis 22.

He started reading the scriptures, and I was taken aback by the number of times God had used the story of Abraham and Sarah to comfort me during whatever trial I was facing in my life at that moment. I reflected on when God told me I would have a son and how each of the plans He laid out for my life came true in His perfect time and place, but the tone of the pastor's voice during this specific sermon was letting me know that this time was different.

> *After these things God tested Abraham and said to him,*
> *"Abraham!" And he said, "Here I am." He said, "Take your*
> *son, your only son Isaac, whom you love, And go to the*
> *land of Moriah, and offer him there as a burnt offering on*
> *one of the mountains of which I shall tell you."*
> Genesis 22:1-2, ESV

As he was reading the scripture, I looked at Brenton with panic in my eyes. I knew this was not the "promise" sermon God had sent before. Pastor warned of a storm that was coming and a hard time that would be at hand. He explained the hard time we would endure was to ultimately bring us closer to God and to his promise that would be waiting on the other side. Yet, all I could think about at the moment was my baby and the fact that this might mean I was going to lose it.

Leaving church that day, I was a broken mess. I remember trying to encourage and convince myself that somehow God meant something else, but I couldn't shake the deep ache in my stomach, swallow the lump in my throat, or slow the rapid pace of my beating heart. Something was coming, and I could feel it in my core.

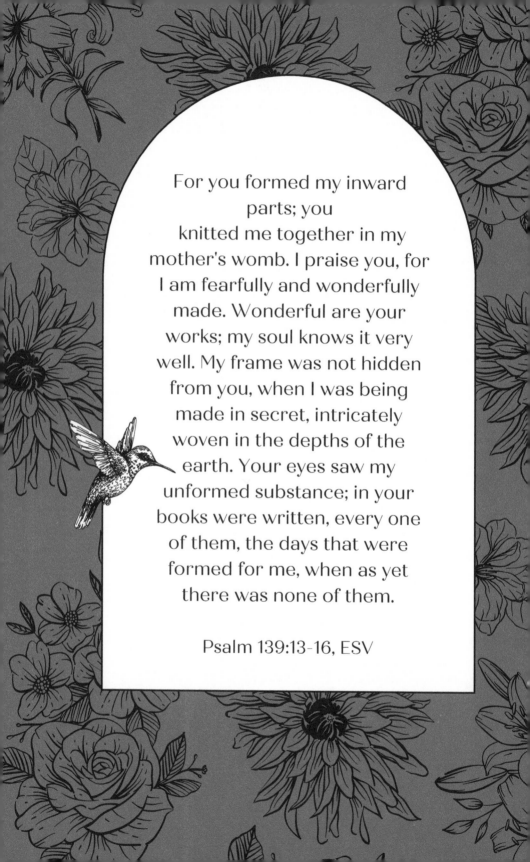

For you formed my inward parts; you knitted me together in my mother's womb. I praise you, for I am fearfully and wonderfully made. Wonderful are your works; my soul knows it very well. My frame was not hidden from you, when I was being made in secret, intricately woven in the depths of the earth. Your eyes saw my unformed substance; in your books were written, every one of them, the days that were formed for me, when as yet there was none of them.

Psalm 139:13-16, ESV

Wednesday morning finally came after weeks of waiting. I was lying on the ultrasound table, holding Brenton's hand, and waiting for the ultrasound tech to come back into the room. She tapped on the door and entered the room. "Okay, let's see this little one," she said and slowly dimmed the lights. I softly prayed to myself the same little chant I had been whispering since I saw the first faint line on the pregnancy test: *Please Lord. Let everything be okay. Please, Lord, don't take this from me.* As I opened my eyes, I looked up at the screen to see a little dark circle and a tiny little peanut coming into view. I felt some relief knowing the little shape of a baby was there, as it should be, but that relief quickly left as the tech remained silent. As a mom of two, I knew the drill; I knew when there was a concern and when everything was okay. She cleared her throat and looked at me with concern in her eyes, "How far along are you?"

My voice quivered as I answered, "Eight and a half weeks."

She nodded and said, "Okay," as she went back to work, measuring and tapping numbers on her keyboard. I was so jittery by this point and my entire body was shaking intensely. She asked me to try to hold still as she kept zooming in on the screen until we clearly saw a tiny little heart beating. She explained I was measuring about two weeks behind, and the heart rate was around seventy bpm, which would be fine for a baby at six weeks because that is when the heart starts to beat for the first time. But, since I was farther along, this might become a concern.

Finishing the appointment, she told me all of the possibilities ahead, considering everything we learned during the ultrasound. She explained a few things I should watch for so I would be aware if I were having a miscarriage. I became angry that she would jump to such conclusions when my baby's heart was indeed beating. I felt her words piercing my faith, so I choked back my words, remained silent, and desperately wanted to be somewhere else. I left the office that day with a heavy heart and an appointment to come back in one week for another ultrasound to remeasure our little baby's growth and to see if its heart rate increased.

Oh, friends, that week was the longest week I ever recall living in my life. I stayed awake at night begging God to allow me to have this child. I asked Him to prove the doubters wrong and show them a true miracle. I was reminded of the woman in the Bible that pressed through the crowd, crawling under many people's feet, just to touch the hem of Jesus' garment. I would have crawled through anything to have a healthy baby. I had complete faith, and I would have done anything to get to Him to save me from the possibilities that engulfed my mind. Yet, I remained helpless, with no healing hem to touch. So, I continued repeating prayers to my Heavenly Father.

I am a fixer by nature, and this was something I couldn't help or fix on my own. All I could do was give it to God, be still, doing nothing, and know He is the only one that can take care of the little innocent life growing inside of me. Every day, hummingbirds appeared in my front windows. I felt as if they were watching my every move, yet I couldn't understand the message they were delivering. I couldn't wrap my mind around the battle I was about to face.

After what felt like two months' time, the follow-up appointment came, and I was back in the office at my next ultrasound staring at that same screen and continually praying for a miracle. As my tiny little baby came into view, I could see the little flicker of its dainty heartbeat. I asked the tech about the bpm. This time, I tried to remain calm, but I was trembling uncontrollably, and Brenton had to help hold my body still so she could gather the measurement. She finally spoke saying, " You should be nine and a half weeks, but the baby has only grown a tiny bit since our last appointment. The heart rate is still below 100." My own heart was beating so quickly. It would have been prime time for a complete heart attack. My worst fear was coming true, and I never felt more helpless in my life. I watched her through a haze of tears in my eyes as she continued to speak, warning me of the things to come. My ears were tuning her voice out completely, as I didn't want to hear any of it. I didn't want to be this person, and the last thing I ever wanted for my life was to be pregnant and helplessly waiting to lose a baby.

As I rode in the passenger seat on the way home, Brenton continually rubbed my hand and asked if I was okay. He tried to encourage me by repeating a few positive facts the nurse had mentioned, but I knew what was coming, and that terrified me. I prayed, yet I felt hopeless. I wanted to believe God would perform this miracle and beat the odds we were against, but I also didn't want to set myself up for worse pain. I kept reflecting on the sermon and the warning of the storm that was coming, and it was evident to me this would be my storm. I knew God was preparing me for the pain I was about to endure, but it didn't make it any easier. There was nothing I could do to heal my unborn baby, and that was all I wanted.

On the Friday after my appointment, I was hosting my niece and nephew for a sleepover. I walked onto the porch to hand out snacks to all of the kiddos, when a hummingbird flew right in front of my face. I flinched back as if it was going to peck my eyeballs right out of my head, but it just hovered in place. I didn't move an inch. I stood completely still, staring into the eyes of the hummingbird as it stared into mine. I felt as if it was gleaming right into the depths of my weary soul. It was so close to my face, I could feel the wind from its tiny wings blowing on my cheeks. After what felt like a few minutes of this intimate encounter, the hummingbird took off and flew straight up into the sky as if it were flying directly into the sun. It continued on until it became a little dot, and that dot became nothing my eyes could see. I knew immediately in my soul, my baby's heart had beat for the last time. At that very moment, I felt light cramping, and that is when my journey of loss began. It was a journey I wasn't prepared for and neither was my heart.

For you formed my inward parts; you knitted me together in my mother's womb. I praise you, for I am fearfully and wonderfully made. Wonderful are your works; my soul knows it very well. My frame was not hidden from you, when I was being made in secret, intricately woven in the depths of the earth. Your eyes saw my unformed substance; in your books were written, every one of them, the days that were formed for me, when as yet there was none of them.
Psalm 139:13-16, ESV

Loss is deep; it's dark, and it's hard. It's lonely and oh-so isolating. You feel as if no one can relate, and you can't escape from the nightmare you wake up to every single morning. It's devastating. I have haunting memories of being in the emergency room bathroom as I was losing my baby. I didn't want to be there, but the doctor had instructed me to go since the miscarriage began after normal office hours. While I was in the bathroom, trying to clean up the floor from the unexpected mess, people were banging on the bathroom door, yelling I was taking too long. I was terrified, and I didn't know what was happening to my body. I had an awful mess all over the bathroom and myself. No one adequately prepared me for what I would need or what would happen when the miscarriage began. I remember crying and wishing I could magically pop myself back home, but I was stuck in my very own nightmare with no way to escape. That night, and the weeks to follow, were the worst in my life as a season of grief took hold of my soul.

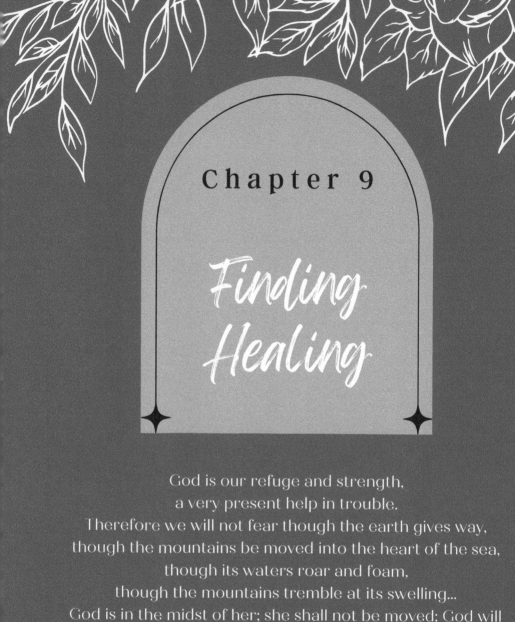

Chapter 9

Finding Healing

God is our refuge and strength,
a very present help in trouble.
Therefore we will not fear though the earth gives way,
though the mountains be moved into the heart of the sea,
though its waters roar and foam,
though the mountains tremble at its swelling...
God is in the midst of her; she shall not be moved; God will
help her when morning dawns... He makes wars cease to
the end of the earth;
He breaks the bow and shatters the spear;
He burns the chariots with fire.
"Be still, and know that I am God."

Psalm 46:1-3,5,9-10, ESV

God is our refuge and strength, a very present help in trouble.
Therefore we will not fear though the earth gives way, though the
mountains be moved into the heart of the sea, though its
waters roar and foam, though the mountains tremble at its swelling...
God is in the midst of her; she shall not be moved; God will help
her when morning dawns... He makes wars cease to the end of
the earth; He breaks the bow and shatters the spear; He
burns the chariots with fire. "Be still, and know that I am God."
Psalm 46:1-3, 5, 9-10, ESV

On August 11, 2017, my sweet baby opened its eyes for the first time to see the face of Jesus.

That moment changed my life forever. I now carried a weight I never knew I could bear. I developed fears I never knew I could have. And I became a person I didn't know I was capable of becoming. The fearless, carefree, laughing-through-the-tears part of me had died and gone with the loss of our baby. I felt the need to tell everyone about my miscarriage because otherwise, this meaningful, tiny life never existed. It was daunting when people would ask me how many kids I have. I would completely freeze and stare at them because I realized the answer would never be correct again. In reality, I knew I had carried three children, but I only held two of them in my arms. My identity had changed completely, and I didn't know how to communicate it to other people.

When we go through loss, we are changed forever, and it is absolutely normal to become a new version of ourselves. We often view those changes as weaknesses, but God wants us to see them as newfound strengths. You are stronger than you ever thought possible to carry a child you never held in

"Therefore we do not lose heart. Though outwardly we are wasting away, yet inwardly we are being renewed day by day. For our light and momentary troubles are achieving for us an eternal glory that far outweighs them all. So we fix our eyes not on what is seen, but on what is unseen, since what is seen is temporary, but what is unseen is eternal."

2 Corinthians 4:16–18, NIV

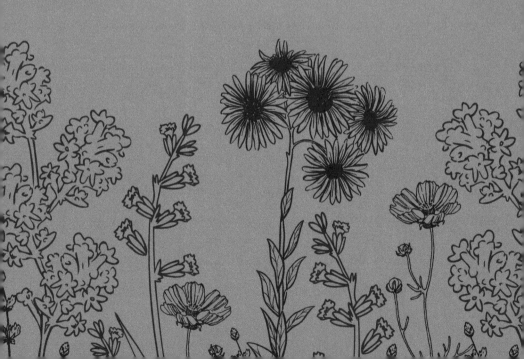

your arms but will stay in your heart forever. I remember miscarriage being my worst fear, and even after going through it, it still is. I never wanted to feel that type of pain, helplessness, and loss. I remember hearing of other mothers going through it and thinking, *Wow, they must be so strong, because if that ever happened to me, I would surely die.* However, once it became a part of my story, I realized what I was capable of through Jesus Christ. He made me strong. He equipped my body to be even stronger, and through this experience, my faith in God became more enduring than ever before.

You might wonder how my faith became stronger when the one thing I fervently prayed for didn't happen. I went through different levels of pain and emotion. I questioned things I never thought I would, and there were two questions I kept asking over and over: *Why did I have to lose my baby? Why do good people have to go through infertility struggles?* The answer I found that gave me the most perspective wasn't an answer but, in fact, another question: *Why was Mary chosen to carry our savior? Can you imagine the burden she carried from the moment she found she was expecting?* She was given a baby and told the baby would grow up to die a cruel death on the cross, to save the entire existence of mankind. Also, she would become pregnant while being a virgin and have to break the news to the love of her life, risking everything. I'm sure she had totally different plans for her life, don't you? I haven't even added the part where she labored on the back of a donkey while traveling miles and miles, finally arriving at an inn without a room for her, and then, she delivered our Savior in a dirty barn full of animals. Wow! I'm feeling pretty amazed by Mary at the moment, aren't you? I mean, I have a barn full of animals, and no matter how much I love farm life, I would never, and I repeat NEVER, give birth in one of my stalls. But what's amazing is the Bible never says Mary freaked out or complained. It never mentions her saying no. She took everything God gave to her and did the best she could. Oh friend, I desperately want to be like that. I want to live with that kind of faith. If you imagined yourself being given a Mary-type task, how would you handle it? What would you do if the Savior was handed to you? Would you be able to carry Him?

"Therefore we do not lose heart. Though outwardly we are wasting

away, yet inwardly we are being renewed day by day. For our light
and momentary troubles are achieving for us an eternal glory that far
outweighs them all. So we fix our eyes not on what is seen, but on what
is unseen, since what is seen is temporary, but what is unseen is eternal."
2 Corinthians 4:16-18, NIV

When I decided to look at my miscarriage as a blessing instead of a curse, my heart became a bit softer. When I saw myself chosen, like Mary, to receive a blessing that was taken from me, I felt an unexpected peace. It doesn't seem fair we have to go through loss and trials in motherhood, but I want to share a few thoughts that gave me comfort during this time in my life.

For everything comes from Him and exists by His power
and is intended for His glory. All glory to Him forever.
Romans 11:36, NLT

This scripture tells us every single thing in this world has been created by God and exists by the power of His mighty hands. He is and always will be the giver of life. No matter how long we try to conceive, follow science, and do as the doctor requests, ultimately, God is the one that knits our bodies together. He decides to give us these little babies we carry, whether it be for a short time or full term. We are blessed to be chosen to carry them at all, and however the story unfolds for us, our journey is ultimately for the glory of God.

"Before I shaped you in the womb, I knew all about you.
Before you saw the light of day, I had holy plans for you:"
Jeremiah 5:1, MSG

When I read these words, it is more evident to me than ever before the value God placed on my unborn baby's life. He had "holy plans," Heavenly plans, for my child. I will never fully comprehend how vast that calling truly is until I'm in heaven. To be "called according to His purpose"[5] upon the first beat of my baby's heart is a special destiny. It's a privilege and not a curse. As I considered these truths, I realized God needed my baby. He needed my innocent, unborn

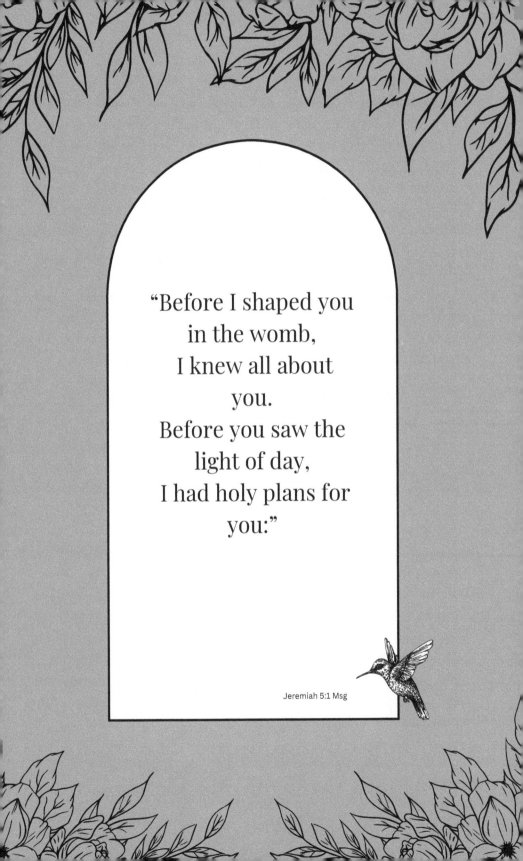

"Before I shaped you
in the womb,
I knew all about
you.
Before you saw the
light of day,
I had holy plans for
you:"

Jeremiah 5:1 Msg

baby, and before that baby saw the light of day, it was called to a greater purpose than anything that could ever be accomplished here on earth. This is the type of gift we can only imagine or dream about. The gift of having a perfect future. My little babe already had a plan for its life, one perfectly mapped out by God, to glorify Him in heaven for every moment of eternity. Pain-free, trial-free, and opening his or her eyes for the first time in awe of Heavenly Perfection. I began to think of my sweet little baby, that God had formed within me, now doing work for my Savior, and I felt a magnitude of peace like never before. I no longer felt like I was cursed, but I felt that I was infinitely *blessed*; blessed to have carried a child, a warrior for God, and the same goes for you. Miscarriage Mommas, we are blessed to be chosen as mothers to more babies than we hold in our arms on this earth. Accepting this truth, restored my faith, and now, I find comfort, instead of anxiety, in knowing how many children I have mothered.

See that you do not despise one of these little ones. For I tell you that in heaven their angels always see the face of my Father who is in heaven.
Matthew 18:10, ESV

Finding Healing

"Be Still and Know" - a song by Hannah Kerr

This song was on repeat as I found my healing. I put a sign over my bed that said, "Be Still and Know." I sang the chorus all day long. I wanted restoration, but there was nothing I could do to fill the void I had within. I just simply needed to know God was holding me. And hold me, He surely did. I felt His presence holding me together like Gorilla Glue, day after day. Otherwise, I surely would have shattered into a million pieces. When the hardest trials come, we must put our trust in Jesus. He has already borne the weight of the world, so there is no burden we face too heavy for Him to bear.

The weeks following my miscarriage were quiet. All signs of hope I had clung to before were gone. Not even a single hummingbird had crossed my path.

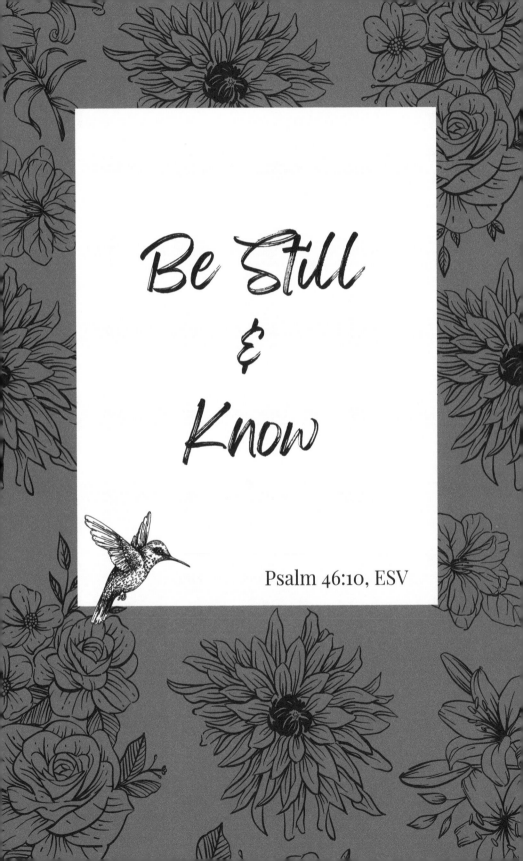

Be Still & Know

Psalm 46:10, ESV

See that you do not despise one of these little ones. For I tell you that in heaven their angels always see the face of my Father who is in heaven.

Matthew 18:10, ESV

Life was still. The stillness is where we find healing, but it is the hardest place to reside. By nature and lifestyle, we are all driven by being busy. If we need something, we can have it here the next day from Amazon. But I assure you, if you search high and low, there is no fix for the deep longing of motherhood on any shopping app or in any store. So, when it comes to a matter of the heart, it is really hard to wait and have your future out of your grasp. Thankfully, God honors patience. He hears our daily cries of desperation, and He is there, whether we notice Him or not.

> *Be Still and know But, in my distress I cried out to the Lord;*
> *Yes, I prayed to my God for help. He heard me from*
> *His sanctuary; my cry to Him reached His ears.*
> Psalm 18:6, NLT

That scripture answers so many questions, am I right? There are multiple times, especially when going through a very hard trial, it feels like you are just praying or pleading, and those prayers are going nowhere. As my mom has said before, "I feel like my prayers are just hitting the ceiling," as if you're just sending them up, and they aren't making it to the Savior. But, this scripture reassures us He is indeed hearing them. Every single one of our cries is reaching His ears. He loves you, He loves me, and He wants healing for our lives.

> *Though He brings grief, He also shows compassion because*
> *of the greatness of His unfailing love. For he does not*
> *enjoy hurting people or causing them sorrow.*
> Lamentations 3:32 & 33, NLT

We see here, God's goal is not to hurt us or harm us but to help us through the struggles or battles we are facing. God understands the pain of losing a loved one because He watched His son die for our sins. He feels our anguish; He is filled with compassion toward us. So, cling to this truth and rip down the barrier you have built between you and God. Accept His compassionate embrace and unfailing love. Fall into His loving arms, and let it all go. We must fully release every burden before true healing begins. We can't heal while we are still hanging onto a load of worries and doubt. Trust that He holds the answer you need and be willing to receive it. He holds our healing and he navigates our motherhood journey, whatever route that may become.

Come to me, all who are weary and burdened, and I will give you rest.
Matthew 11:28, NIV

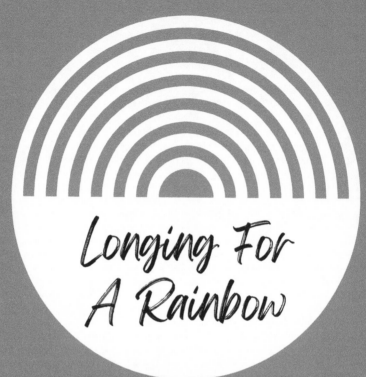

Longing For A Rainbow

Chapter 10

"The best and most beautiful things in the world cannot be seen or touched, but are felt in the heart."-Helen Keller

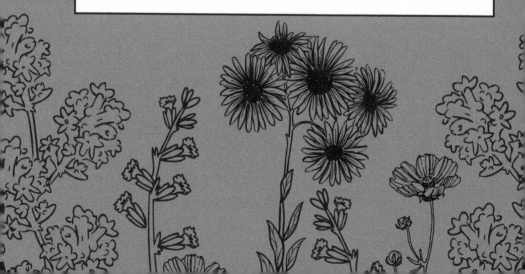

"The best and most beautiful things in the world
cannot be seen or touched, but are felt in the heart."
Helen Keller, author and disability rights advocate (1880–1968)

When God told me to write a book, this is the part of my journey of longing I was living in. I like to call this unknown waiting period longing for a rainbow. This is the moment when you want another baby more than anything. Your thoughts are consumed by it, your diet reflects it, your emotions run deep, and all you can think of is if you are pregnant, will become pregnant, and when that might happen. I have been in the stage of longing for pregnancy. In fact, out of the twelve years of my motherhood journey so far, my fixation years, where I was hoping, praying, and trying to conceive, would be eight out of twelve years. For some, that may seem like a lot of years consumed by longing for motherhood, and for others, that might seem like nothing, as you have been trying for even longer than that. Throughout this season, I felt utterly alone. I felt as if I had no one to talk to because no one had the answer I was looking for.

I felt the only healing that could mend the broken heart I had was to have another baby, to conceive my rainbow baby. I had weathered my storm, I had carried my baby, and now, I desperately needed a rainbow to restore life within my transforming soul. I felt like I lived under the darkest cloud, and even traveling to the warmest sunniest locations didn't escape the decaying death that was consuming the happy version of myself I once was. I had so many thoughts to process, and instead, I just kept pressing them deeper into the back of my mind. This seemed more comfortable than facing all of the layers miscarriage had laid on my life. They were just too painful and extremely overwhelming to sort through.

I remember lying on the couch one rainy day, staring out our front window, as the wind was picking up in the trees. It had been pouring rain for hours, and I felt the weather reflected my mood. As I lay there watching the water spill out of our overfilled gutters and onto my hydrangea bushes, the sky began to brighten up, and the sun started to peek through the dark clouds. The light grew brighter, and the rain still continued to pour from the sky. I quickly got up and ran outside, not even taking a second to slip on shoes. I ran down the porch steps and onto the wet grass. My eyes were wide with anticipation as I searched the entire sky for a rainbow. The rain continued to pour and prayed out loud for a sign that I would find healing soon. I begged God to show himself to me, as I felt the warmth of the sun on my cheeks, but in every angle I looked, the sky was empty. As tears and rain streamed down my face, my prayers turned to screams at God, saying, "SEND ME A RAINBOW!! Show me you will heal my broken heart and never do this to me again!" But there was nothing. Not a single-colored ray of hope. I collapsed onto the saturated ground and sobbed. I was alone. I was hopeless, and I felt like God had utterly abandoned me.

I forced my drenched body from the ground and made my way back to the house. As I walked, I thought about how much I never wanted anyone to have to feel this type of pain. This season of darkness was lonely and isolating; I no longer recognized myself. I needed healing, but I had no idea where to begin without a word or even a sign from God that I would be restored. So I waited on Him, in the stillness.

Behold, I am going to bring to it healing and a remedy, and I will heal them; and I will reveal to them an abundance of peace and truth.
JEREMIAH 33:6, NASB 1995

All praise to the God and Father of our Master, Jesus the Messiah! Father of all mercy! God of all healing counsel! He comes alongside us when we go through hard times, and before you know it, He brings us alongside someone else who is going through hard times so that we can be there for that person just as God was there for us. We have plenty of hard times that

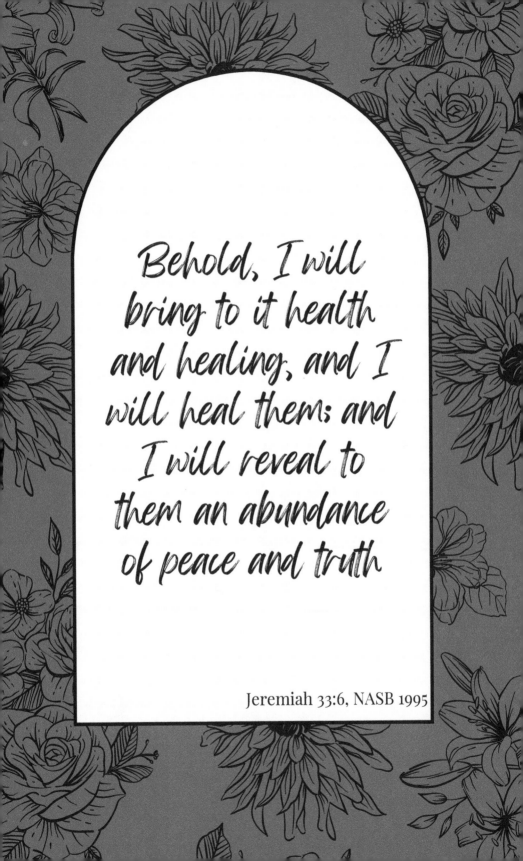

Behold, I will bring to it health and healing, and I will heal them; and I will reveal to them an abundance of peace and truth

Jeremiah 33:6, NASB 1995

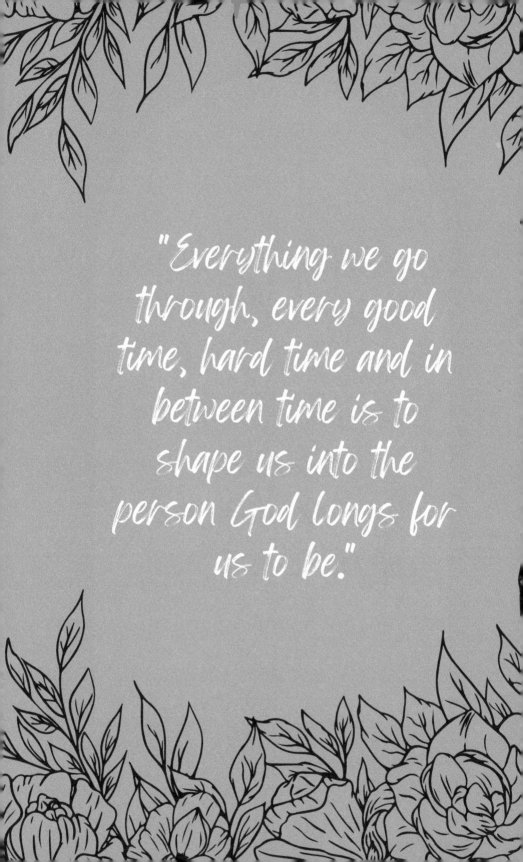

"Everything we go through, every good time, hard time and in between time is to shape us into the person God longs for us to be."

come from following the Messiah, but no more so than the good times of
His healing comfort- we get a full measure of that, too.
2 Corinthians 1:3-5, MSG

After a few months, I felt one way I could find healing was to give my baby a voice and to give other mothers' babies a voice as well. As the fall season approached, I decided to tell the world about our miscarriage. I shared the painful story I have now shared with you on my blog. At the end of the blog post, I gave an invitation for other mothers to confide in me with their stories of loss so I could share the burden they had been carrying alone, to tell me of the lives they lost too soon, and of the babies they never got to hold in their arms. My inbox filled quickly with friends who had been through this pain, and I never knew. Young women confided in me the losses they had endured. Some of my friends' mothers sent me the stories they had held deep in their hearts, bearing them alone for years upon years, never telling a soul. Grandmothers even called me. They told me about their lost babies from fifty years ago, a painful experience and secret they held onto for all of that time. My ear was bleeding. My heart was broken for their losses, and I shared a heavy burden with them. But through this, I realized my purpose, and I knew I was no longer alone.

Each of the women gave me the strength I desperately needed, a fighting purpose, a sense of belonging, and a voice for our unborn babies that were no longer in secret. The sins of this earth are the reason for the battles that involve losing someone we love so deeply. The Bible says that the trials we face sadden God, but they all work together for His good. I want you to ask yourself: What is your purpose? And how has the battle or detour your life's journey has taken impacted that purpose?

To the woman He said:
"I will greatly multiply your sorrow and your
conception; In pain you shall bring forth children;"
Genesis 3:16, NKJV

This is the reason we go through our losses. This is the purpose of every strife we face on this earth. Suffering was never God's plan for our lives, which is why it pains Him so deeply to watch us endure these trials. He designed the perfect world we so desire in Genesis chapter one. This was the plan he ultimately wanted for His children, but because of the sin of Eve and Adam, we all experience the sorrow they caused. Knowing this fact alone should remove any blame you place on yourself for the losses you endure.

Your labor sufferings are not your fault, and the ending result will never be in your control since God is the Author of our existence. There is nothing you could possibly do to change the result of the maternal battle you have fought or are fighting.

Everything we go through, every good time, hard time, and in-between time, is to shape us into the person God longs for us to be. This person is to glorify God in every way possible. So, ask yourself today, what might that purpose be? What might God want to do with your life tomorrow that requires this difficult journey today? There is no right or wrong answer to that question. Though our battles might be similar, each of us has something unique to take away from it, a different lesson to learn, and a specific destiny set before us. Vow today not to let that hard time go to waste. Let God do a magnificent change in your life, build your character, and mold you into a better version of yourself from the struggles you've endured. A stronger, braver you. Look in the mirror, and know that you are loved, you are called, and you have a powerful purpose through Jesus Christ.

My prayer for you is this:

Dear Loving God,
I pray today you send healing and direction, shine a light where
there is darkness, and place insight where there is blindness.
I ask you to reveal the purpose of the battles you have placed on
our lives. Give us guidance to use these struggles for your glory.
Remove loneliness and isolation during the stillness, Give
us a sense of unity, one to another, and mend broken hearts.

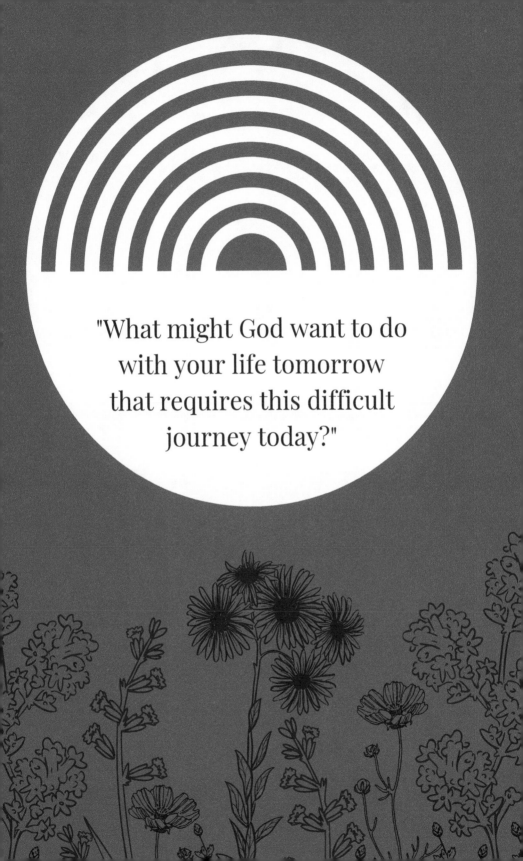

"What might God want to do
with your life tomorrow
that requires this difficult
journey today?"

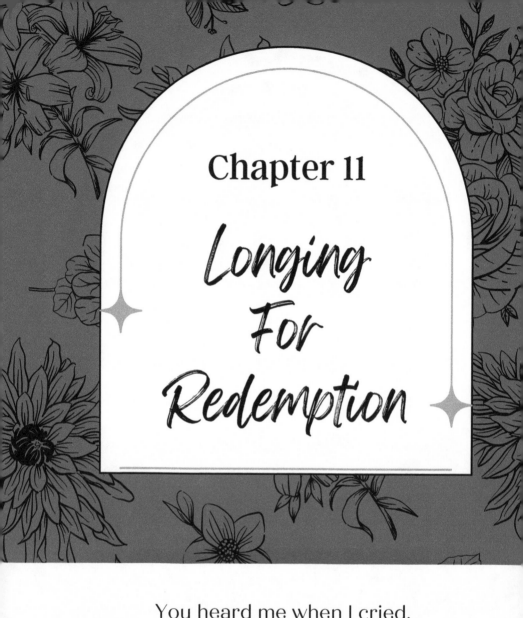

Chapter 11

Longing For Redemption

You heard me when I cried,
"Listen to my pleading! Hear my cry for help!"
Yes, You came when I called; You told me,
"Do not fear." Lord, You have come to my
defense; You have redeemed my life.

Lamentations 3:56-58, NLT

"An estimated 23 million miscarriages occur every year worldwide, translating to 44 pregnancy losses each minute."[6]

We are NOT Alone.

It had been a long, cold winter. The darkness continued to make its appearance every evening around 4:30, and I felt as if that same darkness was encapsulating my heart a little more with each passing day. I longed for a third child. My soul ached for healing, and my dimming heart desperately needed the redemption of our rainbow baby. After months of trying to conceive without success, I was beginning to wonder if my story would end like this. Would I live in this position forever? Would my body conceive again? I felt broken, and I was quickly losing hope that my dream of having four kids would ever become a reality.

As much as I prayed in this silent season, all of the signs of hope God had used prior to the miscarriage were gone. Not a single sermon on Abraham and Sarah in the passing months, not a single hummingbird had crossed my path or fluttered past my living room window. (Although, I had prayed to God that he would never show me a sign related to pregnancy through a hummingbird again after using the last one through loss.) It was the most silent season I had ever experienced in my relationship with God.

"Jesus called out with a loud voice, ...
"My God, My God, why have you abandoned me?""
Matthew 27:46, NLT

We see in this scripture Jesus questioned God, asking why He abandoned Him. This should reassure our souls as we realize even Jesus felt isolated. In

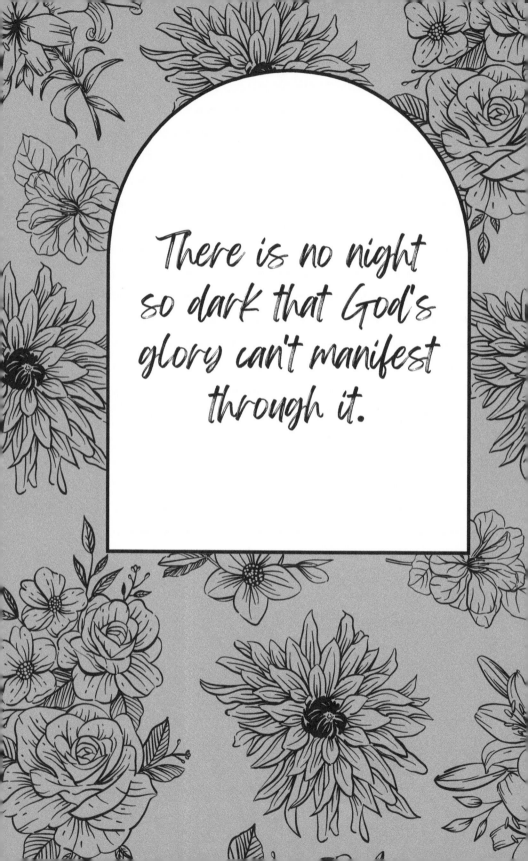

There is no night so dark that God's glory can't manifest through it.

fact, for every type of pain we'll ever endure, Jesus has already taken for us on the cross. Have you ever been through a season like this? Maybe you are here now, and it's hard to continue to pray through the silence. But God wants us to seek after Him, even when we can't hear His reply or sense the return of His embrace. Do as Jesus did, keep the faith, and cling to the word He has already given. He still hears us, and through those prayers, we are developing a stronger relationship with Him.

As the end of winter approached, I hit my breaking point. I prayed to God and told Him I was done. I couldn't do this anymore. I couldn't carry this burden while trying for another child. In my own strength, I was constantly trying, trying to grow closer to Him, trying to be perfect enough to deserve another child, trying to be healthy enough to conceive. It was exhausting, and I was tapping out.

"Father, if you are willing,
please take this cup of suffering away from me.
Yet I want your will to be done, not mine." [13]
Luke 22:42, NLT

Jesus felt exhaustion and fear when He was looking at the cross. He prayed for hours asking God to let the suffering pass from Him. He "asked," yet He remained sinless. This tells us, it's okay to feel the many layers that loss and longing bring into our lives. But it's what we do with them that really matters. We see how Jesus asked but still, He said, "Yet, I want your will to be done, not mine." He fully believed this. He had complete faith in God's ultimate plan for His destiny and the effects it would also have on ours. We must also keep the faith. God doesn't want our perfection; He wants our truth, our realness, and our faithfulness to Him, no matter how hard the journey looks ahead. I wish I had understood the beauty of God's love during those hard times. God didn't want my "TRY" the way I thought He did. He just wanted my faith. He wanted an unshakable faith in Him that no matter what I felt at the moment, I trusted He was working behind the scenes for a better future.

Then Abraham fell on his face and laughed and said to himself,
"Shall a child be born to a man that is a hundred years old?
Shall Sarah, who is ninety years old, bear a child?" ... God said, "No but Sarah
your wife shall bear you a son and you shall call him Isaac. I will establish my
covenant with him as an everlasting covenant for his offspring after him.
Genesis 17:17 & 19, NIV

We see Abraham question and doubt God in this scripture, yet even through His questions, God assured Abraham He would indeed deliver the promise in the timing He had established. Sometimes in life, just when we are ready to jump off the cliff, God is there to catch us. When we reach the point when we are so completely exhausted of our own options, we are fully ready to hand over everything to God. That's when He will fully take control of our lives and show us what He can do with them. Oh, but if only we, as humans, were capable of letting go of the reins before we reach that point of desperation before we reach that point of darkness and depletion. And maybe you can, but I know for me, it's been hard to fully and completely let go and let God take over my life without holding onto something. Thankfully, there is no night so dark that God's glory can't manifest through it.

The Lord said, "I will surely return to you about this
time next year, and Sarah your wife shall have a son."
Genesis 18:10, NIV

I found myself in a familiar position, one I had been in over and over again. Month after month, pretty much for the past three and half years. Sitting on a cold white toilet seat staring at a pregnancy test and waiting for the pink line to appear. As I sat there, a million possibilities and scenarios flooded my mind. Like, how would I feel if my redemption was in my hands this time? Or what would I do if another month passes by without my rainbow? As I gazed into my palms, slowly the first line started to come into view. As the watermark made its way to the end of the stick, I saw what appeared to be a second faint line coming into view. My heart rate doubled as it was becoming more obvious that this test was positive, and I was holding a sure sign of a rainbow in

"God doesn't want our perfection; He wants our truth, our realness, and our faithfulness to Him no matter how hard the journey looks ahead."

my hands. I burst into tears as I prayed, "Thank you, God" over and over. My deliverance was coming, and I would no longer be a slave to this storm that was placed on my life.

The next few days, I took a completely normal amount of pregnancy tests. (Insert many laughing emojis, because I think you know me well enough to know, which means enough to fill an entire bathroom drawer.) I was trying to ease my fears, and even though the tests were all dark, with obvious positive double lines and plus signs, my heart was changed. I had fears I hadn't had with my other two children because I knew my body had failed me before. I knew I was capable of miscarriage, and I wasn't sure if God had that in his plans for me once more.

On the Sunday after I found out I was pregnant, my little family of four made our way to church. Brenton and I sat in our same row, and Bentley and Baize sat right with us, as they always do. I had a joy in my heart I hadn't felt in months and a weight on my shoulders I couldn't quite explain. As our pastor began to read from the Bible, the scriptures rang a very familiar tune. "The Lord visited Sarah as He had said, and the Lord did to Sarah as He had promised. And Sarah conceived and bore Abraham a son in his old age at the time of which God had spoken to him" (Genesis 20:1-2, NIV). My eyes instantly locked with Brenton's and I began to cry. I actually cried the entire sermon as our pastor spoke about God's promises and faithfulness. God shows up on time, in His own perfect timing, right when you think he might have forgotten you. I felt His redemption covering me like a blanket. This was for me. This was where my story would change. I felt His redeeming love flooding into my life as my silent period was over. I knew this child was promised to me and would be our rainbow baby.

I want you to know that the stories we read in the Bible are still happening today. People still receive healing. Miracles still happen, and I have seen several in my thirty-five years on this earth. Whatever comes to mind when you think of a miracle for yourself, it is not too hard for God. He is still willing and able to provide a way when you think there is none. The hard part, that most

Don't cover up
your flaws,
brokenness, and
exhaustion when
pleading at the
cross.

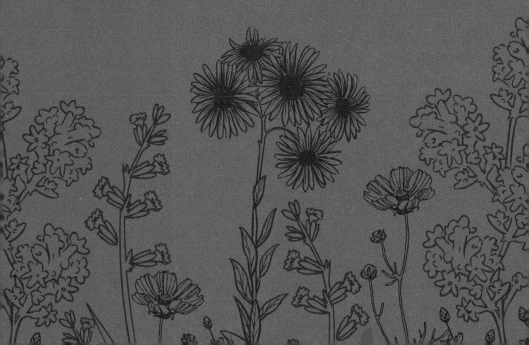

people miss when asking and waiting for God's plan, is understanding that sometimes it doesn't come exactly as you think or want. We have to come to that place of desperation, letting go of all control, and completely letting God take the reins of our life. We must be willing to receive the precise plans God has for our lives, even when it's not the exact path we had in mind. When our plans align with God's journey, peace is attainable through Him.

Even Abraham and Sarah had a season of doubt. Towards the end of Sarah's forty years trying for a baby, she gave up on God ever giving her a son to carry on Abraham's lineage, so much so, she arranged for her maid to become pregnant by him instead (Say what now, sister??). Yes, what you read is true, and we see it in the scriptures here:

> *Sarai, Abram's wife, hadn't yet produced a child.*
> *She had an Egyptian maid named Hagar. Sarai said*
> *to Abram, "God has not seen fit to let me have a child.*
> *Sleep with my maid. Maybe I can get a family from her."*
> Genesis 16:1-2, MSG

Wow! That's some serious doubt and desperation! Now, how do you think this plan of Sarah's (then named Sarai) played out? If you guessed it ended terribly, you are correct! She gave up right before we see God giving her the promise of her very own son. In an act of desperation, she took matters into her own hands, which ultimately caused her grief for the rest of her life. Oh, Sarah ... If you could only see what we see. You would have known that your timing just wasn't right, and God's plan was only a few years from the moment He gave you the true longings of your heart.

The lesson we can learn from this part of Sarah's story is the value of waiting on God while not losing faith in Him. He always has a conclusive plan for our lives, even when His timing isn't our own agenda. Do you see now how disastrous things can end when he allows us to make choices for our own lives? He *will* allow us to make our own decisions and experience the grief those choices will bring to our lives. This is why we must give Him complete control of our circumstances because He is the only all-knowing One that can see the futuristic result.

We also need to acknowledge what a picture of God's love this is as her story unfolds. Sarah grew desperate from waiting on God and worked out a plan of her very own, and she experienced the consequences of that plan forever. BUT, God never held that over her and still gave her a son of her very own. Oh my, do you see how much this shows the magnitude of God's love for His children? He continually gives what we don't deserve. So ... Just like the place I was in before I found out I was pregnant with our third child, I had no strength left in me. I was done, and it was at that point, I was able to let go and then see the glory of God go to work in my life like I never had before. But, what do you think might have happened if I had taken matters into my own hands, or grown weary from the journey, lost hope, and walked away from my faith in God? Oh, friend, I don't even want to think about how disastrous my life might have become.

Ultimately, God wants a relationship with you, my dear friend. He wants you to pray to Him, ask miracles of Him, need Him, and WAIT for Him. He wants us to be real in the good times and also the bad. Don't cover up your flaws, brokenness, and exhaustion when pleading at the cross. Let Him see it all. Depend on him, have faith in Him, and fully lean into His fatherly embrace. It's there, at that moment, when true redemption begins to take place.

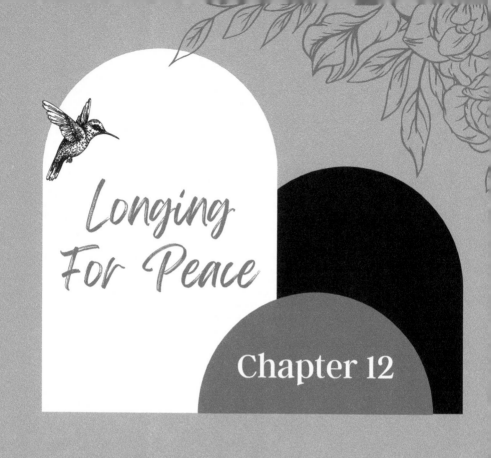

Longing For Peace

Chapter 12

True peace doesn't rest within our circumstances. True peace comes through prayer, laying our burdens down at Jesus' feet, and completely falling into our Father's arms.

True peace doesn't rest within our circumstances.
True peace comes through prayer,
laying our burdens down at His feet,
and completely falling into our Father's arms.

Life after loss is an emotionally dark road to travel. After experiencing the trauma of miscarriage, it was impossible to erase those haunting memories from my mind. I recall my doctor suggesting not to have a D&C and to let my body pass our baby on its own. I thought this was a good idea, however, I also didn't realize for the next six weeks, I would be continuously losing our baby in a toilet or in pads. Miscarriage for me came as laboring contractions and was followed by a massive hemorrhage, over and over for weeks. Unexpected floods while working, or standing in line at a store, resulted in a mad dash to the car and a phone call to my husband for a change of clothes. Many times thereafter, I'd sit locked in my car, trying to sort through the stream of emotions I endured alone. These are the things no one speaks about. These are the moments we keep to ourselves, that continually haunt our dreams and convince us that we are crazy. Moments like these completely change you forever.

My soul, wait in silence for God alone, for my hope is from Him.
He alone is my rock and my salvation, my refuge; I will not be shaken.
Psalm 62:5-6, NASB

Finding healing comes in different forms, unique to each person's circumstances. The Bible says: "God is our refuge, a very pleasant help during trouble" (Psalm 46:1, NIV). This scripture remains true. If you think about it, God also lost his son. He has been through the most excruciating pain as He watched His son grow through perfection, witnessed the world turn against him, then watched him die a cruel death to save the ones who betrayed Him

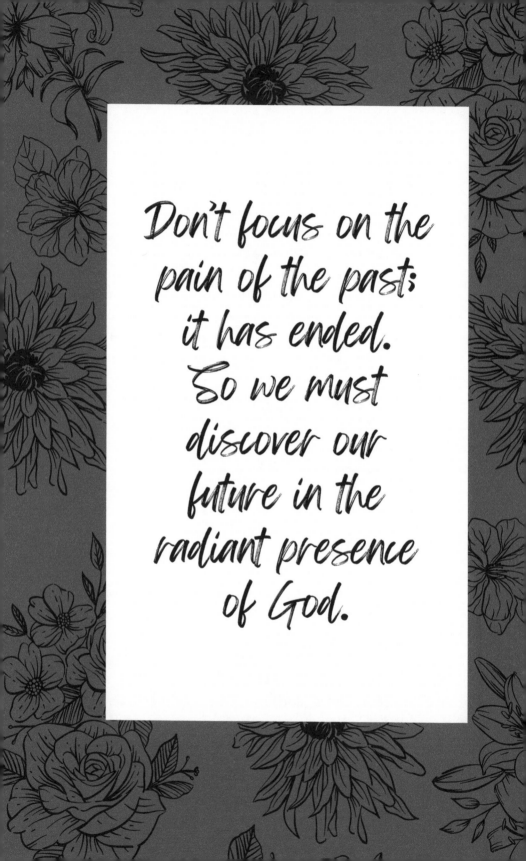

Don't focus on the pain of the past; it has ended. So we must discover our future in the radiant presence of God.

and the entire world thereafter. So He knows the pain of loss, and He also knows how deeply we need peace to find healing.

Healing comes in many forms. I thought my pregnancy with our rainbow baby would bring all of the healing I longed for, but my spirit remained uneasy. I worried daily I would lose her too. Each cramp, backache, and spot sent me into a spiral of emotion and fear. Knowing the possibilities and the memories of the things I had encountered, woke me up in a panic during the night. I was on the way to healing, but I was lacking peace.

A step towards finding peace comes with closure from the pain of your past. I have found that constantly reflecting on the trauma I had been through and the pain loss brought to me, set me back in that same place over and over again. I wasn't able to feel at peace because the memories and fears I played in my mind weren't allowing me to. I needed closure.

Closure after a miscarriage is hard to find because most women never get to physically see their baby to be able to say goodbye. The baby never lived outside of your womb, and it is taken almost as soon as it was given. Closure, though, can be found in many different forms. Some might receive a special piece of jewelry, name a star, or get a significant tattoo. I thought about the things I felt would give me peace in the memory of my lost baby, and I decided I would plant a magnolia tree. My plan for this tree was to watch each limb as it grew, reaching closer to the sky with each passing year. I wanted to find peace in its growth, a symbol of the life that was taken too soon from me. It, in many ways, gave revival to my soul. Another way I found closure was through supporting a mission. I decided to adopt a child to support each month through Compassion International. This gave me a sense of having another child to care for without actually knowing them or physically seeing them and caring for them. These two things helped me feel like I had closure, but ultimately, the most amazing peace is found in God. He has witnessed more pain and suffering than any human being on earth. He has mended millions of broken hearts and restored empty souls.

And after you have suffered a little while, the God of grace,
who has called you to his eternal glory in Christ, Will
himself restore, confirm, strengthen and establish you.
1 Peter 5:10, ESV

When I read those words, I see God's promise that today's sufferings won't last a lifetime. However, when we are in the midst of the storm at hand, it's hard to look ahead to the future and find peace in uncertainties. BUT, this is why we must not look around for our comforts. True peace doesn't lie within our circumstances, whether they are good or bad. True peace is held in our Father's arms. So, when you feel out of control or that all of the darkness is closing in, just look up! Don't focus on everyday tasks. Don't focus on the pain of the past; it has ended. So, we must discover our future in the radiant presence of God. We must place all of our worries and cares on Him, and focus on Him and only Him. Today won't last forever, and yesterday is now gone. So, I want to find peace in knowing that tomorrow will be better.

Do not be anxious about anything, but in everything by prayer
and supplication with thanksgiving let your request be made known
to God. And the peace of God, which surpasses all understanding,
will guard your hearts and your minds in Jesus Christ.
Philippians 4:6-7, ESV

Through this Scripture, we find comfort in knowing God's promise of peace. When you feel uneasy, pray. When you feel emotions overwhelming you, pray. If you can't seem to find the answer, pray. God is telling us here in all of our circumstances and with all of our thoughts, we should take them to Him through prayer. In our daily lives, it can be difficult to think this way. It seems easier to let our negative thoughts consume us as we try to find something we can "do" about the problems we are facing. However, the continual worry of our minds only allows us to "feel" like we are helping ourselves, while the reality is, worrisome thoughts help nothing. This is where anxiety creeps in, our thoughts run out of control, and peace becomes unattainable.

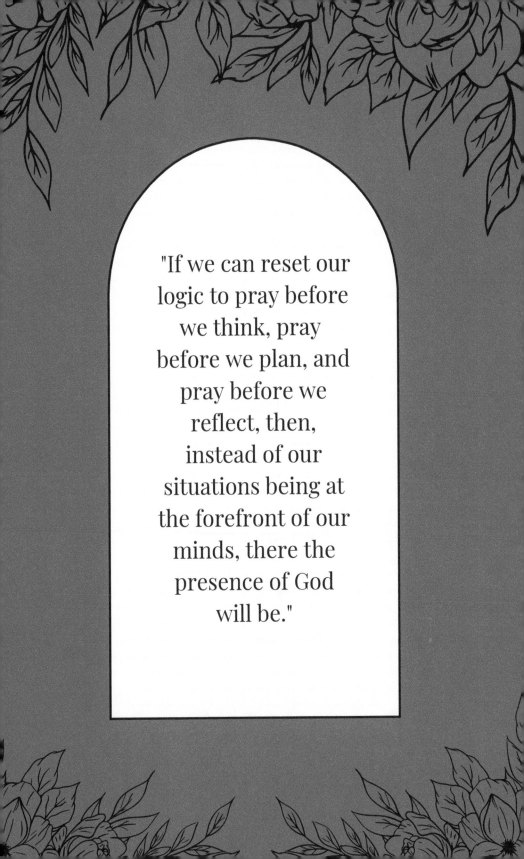

"If we can reset our logic to pray before we think, pray before we plan, and pray before we reflect, then, instead of our situations being at the forefront of our minds, there the presence of God will be."

"It seems so much easier to let our negative thoughts consume us as we try to find something we can "do" about the problems we are facing. However, the continual worry of our minds only allows us to "feel" like we are helping ourselves while the reality is, worrisome thoughts help nothing."

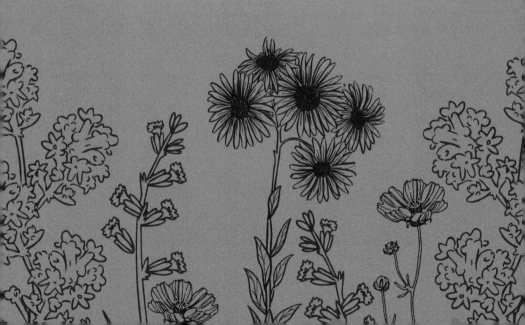

If we can reset our logic to pray before we think, pray before we plan, and pray before we reflect, then, instead of our situations being at the forefront of our minds, there the presence of God will be. In God's presence, we can view our surroundings with a clearer mindset and vision, while allowing the peaceful spirit of God to flood our souls.

Open your heart today and allow His peace to enter. Hand over the burden that has been weighing you down. I have found when I keep a tight grip on my problems, that's all I can seem to focus on. Release the tight grasp you have on your life, and through prayer, reset your mind and truly find peace today.

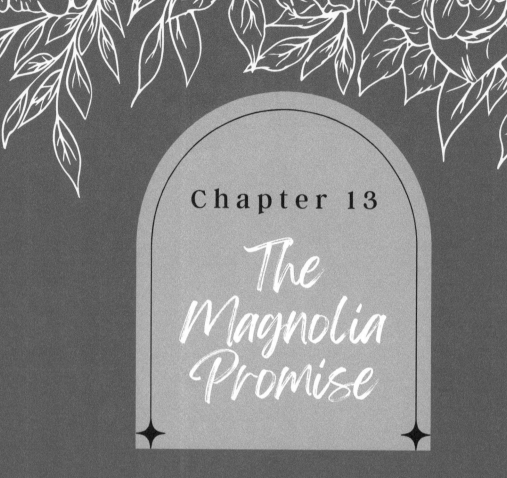

Chapter 13

The Magnolia Promise

For you formed my inward parts; you knitted me together in my mother's womb. I praise you, for I am fearfully and wonderfully made. Wonderful are your works; my soul knows it very well. My frame was not hidden from you, when I was being made in secret, intricately woven in the depths of the earth. Your eyes saw my unformed substance; in your books were written, every one of them, the days that were formed for me, when as yet there was none of them.

Psalm 139:13-16 ESV

For you formed my inward parts; you knitted me together in my mother's womb. I praise you, for I am fearfully and wonderfully made. Wonderful are your works; my soul knows it very well. My frame was not hidden from you, when I was being made in secret, intricately woven in the depths of the earth. Your eyes saw my unformed substance; in your books were written, every one of them, the days that were formed for me, when as yet there was none of them.
Psalm 139:13-16, ESV

Through the birth of our precious rainbow baby came healing and restoration of my soul that I thought might never take place. The very moment they placed her in my arms, I felt a revival occur in my darkened heart. There was light in my life where the darkness had taken over, and joy now lived where uncertainty had dwelled for so long. We named her Beacon Meadow. She was a Beacon to me in one of the hardest storms I had ever faced, and Meadow reminded me of the peace I felt in my heart when my mind was overwhelmed with grief. When you think of a meadow, it always seems peaceful, don't you think? As the wind blows in a meadow, the tops of the long grassy stems lean and sway back and forth. It's mesmerizing. When I say her name, it has meaning and purpose. Although I don't go a day without thinking of the baby I lost, I felt I wouldn't continue to live under the dark cloud I had been stuck under.

It's crazy how life after loss changes the way you think. I view myself as a survivor now, as I do all mothers who have been through loss. We have battle scars, and we have continued on being strong for our other children and husbands that depend on us every single day.

rainbow baby: a baby born subsequent to a miscarriage, stillbirth, or the death of an infant from natural causes.[7]

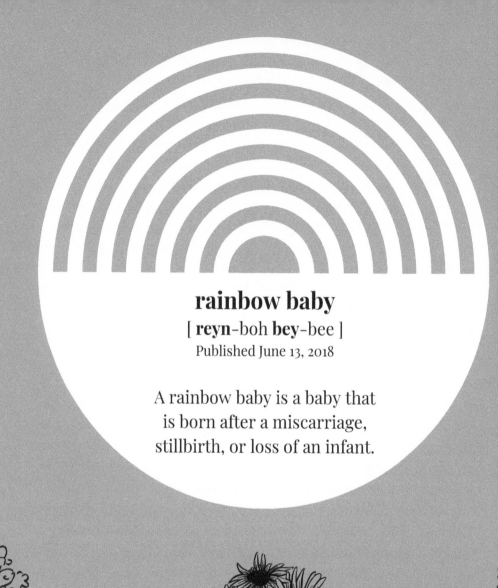

rainbow baby

[**reyn**-boh **bey**-bee]

Published June 13, 2018

A rainbow baby is a baby that
is born after a miscarriage,
stillbirth, or loss of an infant.

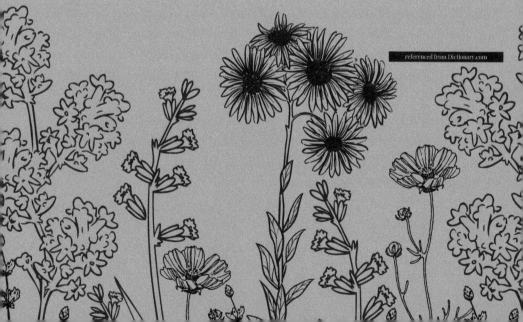

The term "rainbow baby" was added to "dictionary.com" in 2018. Since then, it has become widely used amongst mothers through social media platforms, online parenting forums, and real-life conversations. For years, the subject of miscarriage has been an unspoken topic, but through the term "rainbow baby," mothers were able to announce their pregnancy while also giving tribute to the baby they carried and lost.

When I think of a rainbow, my mind automatically goes to the story of Noah's Ark in the Bible. Surely, I'm not alone in this thought. This is the story of the very first rainbow, which was a promise from God to Noah, and all people, He would never flood the entire earth again. Every time it rains and the sun begins to shine at the same time, we get to see God's miraculous, colorful paintings in the sky, and we are reminded of that wonderful promise all over again. When I put that same promise in terms of my loss, I felt sure I would never experience a miscarriage again, but unfortunately, that's not always the way it goes. Sometimes, people go through loss once, twice, or even more times. I can't begin to wrap my mind around that possibility nor fathom how I would survive that type of pain over and over again. I can't tell you why that would happen to any one person because, in every way I look at it, it just seems unfair. This is where our faith comes in. We must have faith that God's plan is much greater than the plans we have for our own lives.

Shortly after Beacon's second birthday, Brenton and I began talking about what our family would look like if we were never able to have four kids. We knew how blessed we were to already have three healthy children and how difficult it was to become pregnant with each one of them. We also knew how deeply it hurt to lose a baby and never wanted to experience that type of pain again. We spent many nights talking about going back to the fertility clinic, but we felt guilty for wanting another child when we had already experienced God's miracles three times before. After re-examining the last two years without conceiving, in an act of desperation, we decided to make the appointment. This time we hoped for a procedure so we could have a better chance of becoming pregnant one last time. In order to have a procedure done at the clinic, you must have your menstrual cycles charted and on a regular schedule. I was

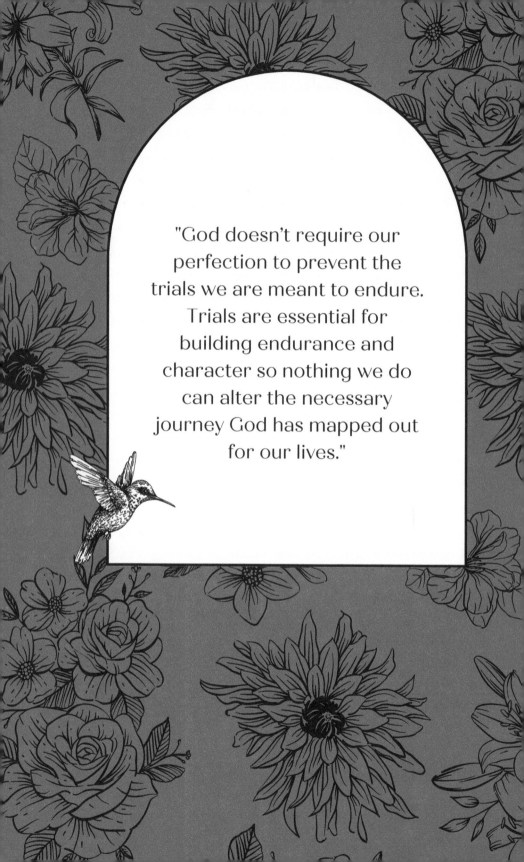

"God doesn't require our perfection to prevent the trials we are meant to endure. Trials are essential for building endurance and character so nothing we do can alter the necessary journey God has mapped out for our lives."

pretty much always on a regular schedule, so I didn't see this causing any delays.

On the morning of my appointment, the air was crisp, the leaves were turning, and I was wearing my favorite sweater. All of my favorite things were telling me it would be a good day. As I drove my car down the driveway, I glanced out the window to see my little magnolia tree as I did every single day for the past four years. This little tree had remained the same shape since the day I placed it in the ground. It hadn't grown a single inch and not a single bloom had ever budded from its branches. Like most of my perfect plans, this little tree had pretty much been the opposite of a symbol of life for our lost baby. Still, every day, I searched for a little change, the slightest bit of growth from its limbs. Yet, just like the days prior, today was the same. On the way to the fertility clinic, signs of fall were around me, and that instantly put me in a good mood (well, that and jamming to my favorite Britt Nicole playlist). I just knew it was going to be a good day, and I couldn't wait to have a plan in place to have our last baby. From the moment my appointment began, I assured the doctor my recent menstrual cycles had been on time and that I would be ready for a procedure the next month. He knew the details of the issues we encountered while trying to conceive before, so he agreed to get me in and waste no time with the normal, required testing. As we finished our appointment, he said, "So, looking at your menstrual cycle schedule, you should have started yesterday?" Then, looking up from his papers, he asked, "Did you?" Well, I'm sure I looked five kinds of puzzled because, for the first time in a very long time, I hadn't realized I was actually two days late. I quickly put a confident smile on my face and answered with a nervous jitter in my voice, "No ... ummm ... but I'm sure I will today."

On the drive home, I couldn't believe I had not realized I was a couple of days late for my period. With all of the anticipation around this appointment, I hadn't even noticed I had not started yet. This was huge for me because I am always well aware of when I am late. I usually have a big Amazon bag of tests, and I'm ready at any given moment to take one. This day, however, was different. I was completely caught by surprise, and my last test was taken the month before. Now, I'm sure you can guess my first stop right after leaving the doctor's office, and if not, I'll tell you, it was the good ole' Dollar General to purchase whatever kind of test they had available. As soon as I got home, I practically ran to the bathroom. By this point, my nerves were shredded, and my stomach was in knots. As I sat there, I closed my eyes tight, then slowly opened them to see the pregnancy test with two light pink lines. My heart was beating so hard I could feel it in my throat. I stared at the positive test in my hands. I felt the lines should be darker considering how far along I would be at this point in pregnancy. Tears filled my eyes, and I began to cry. Call it a mother's intuition, but this time was different, and I felt something was wrong.

Over the next few days, I took a lot of pregnancy tests. I'm pretty sure I took every brand on the market, and every time, I prayed and begged God to make the lines darker, but each day, they were fading away little by little. I felt my baby slipping from me before I even got to be excited about carrying it, and there was nothing I could do about it.

When I was six weeks pregnant, our baby saw the face of Jesus, and I lost a part of me I will never get back. The pain I felt with this miscarriage was so much deeper than the one I'd had before. This time, I was mourning both of the pregnancies I lost and that I would never hold either of those babies in my arms. They wouldn't be able to feel my touch or know how much I loved them. They would never have a voice, and the deep pain I felt was in silence because no one knew. No one knew I was a mother of five babies since two of them were never carried full term. My identity changed again that day, and I didn't know if the carefree version of myself I once was would ever be attainable. This caused me to question God, and I wondered why I had to go through this, not only once, but another time. I never wanted to experience the pain of losing a baby, so why would He do this to me twice? I had surrendered every area of my life I thought was possible to surrender.

Even before he made the world, God loved us and chose
us in Christ to be holy and without fault in his eyes.
Ephesians 1:4, NLT

Even before He made the world, God loved us and chose us in Christ to be holy and without fault in His eyes.

Ephesians 1:4, NLT

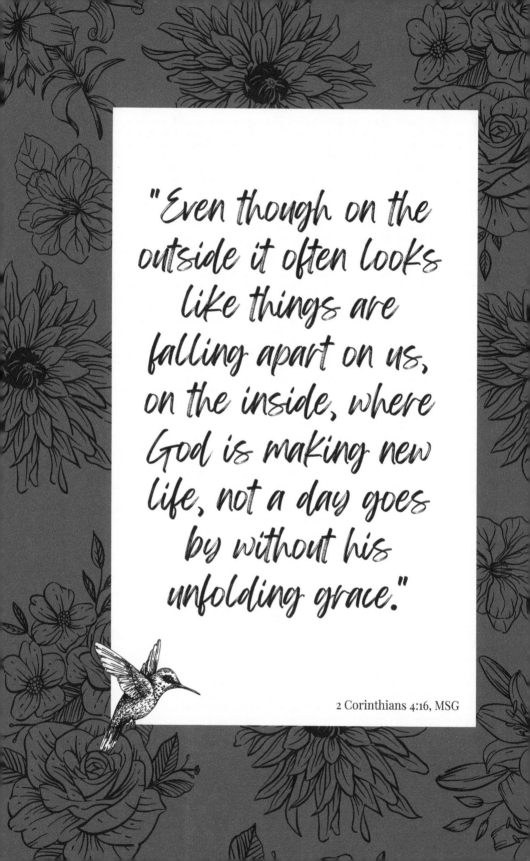

"Even though on the outside it often looks like things are falling apart on us, on the inside, where God is making new life, not a day goes by without his unfolding grace."

2 Corinthians 4:16, MSG

I, yet again, tried to live a perfect life that would be pleasing to God. I had already shared our story of how He worked miracles, how He took our baby and then gave us a rainbow baby, through my blog. I had forgotten God doesn't require our perfection to prevent the trials we are meant to endure. Trials are essential for building endurance and character so nothing we do can alter the necessary journey God has mapped out for our lives. Unfortunately, I pushed myself as I tried to live in perfection and do every single thing God led me to do while hoping to prevent this pain from ever happening again to me. Yet, there I sat, arms full of three children and darkness in my heart. I couldn't communicate with anyone. I felt guilty for being sad when I had three other blessings he has given me. I had multiple people, very close friends, tell me to let the dream of more kids go and be happy with what I had. Those words stung my heart, and they told me I was wrong. The empty advice from others desperately trying to say the right thing convinced me I was crazy, and I was grieving alone.

I prayed and begged God to show up in my life in a mighty way. I needed to know He was there. I needed to know He still loved me, and I wasn't alone. A few days after my second miscarriage, I was driving up the driveway. I looked out the car window to see my little magnolia tree like I had every other day, but this time, it was different. It looked like there were little flowers budding on it. I stopped the car and walked over to get a better look. As I got closer, I started to count the buds. One, two, three... I felt God's love wrapping around me. Four, Five... My heart was beating so fast as I searched for one more, and there, in the back, was number six. The sweetest little bloom. I felt God speaking to me and saying, "These are your promises, five for each of your babies you've carried, and one more for the one you will conceive." At that moment, I felt His redemption. I felt His love for me. Even though I was still living in the darkness of loss and mourning, at that moment, I was given hope for the future.

Later the next week, I received a call from the clinic. We had been waiting on the results of Brenton's analysis the doctor had required the week before. The lady's voice on the other end of the phone was kind yet hesitant. She explained the results of the test he'd had and apologized as she delivered the news that we wouldn't be candidates for any type of procedure to help us get pregnant. She explained that if we decided to try again on our own, each time would end in a miscarriage, and the doctor did not advise it. I questioned how sure he was and if what she was telling me was that we would never have another baby, and she responded with, "I'm so sorry, but yes; that's exactly what I'm telling you." At that moment, it was all I could do not to burst into a million pieces. So many thoughts flooded my mind as the tears streamed down my face. I didn't understand why this would be happening to us. I questioned God. Wasn't losing two babies enough? I felt I would never recover from this pain without the redemption of another child. I knew the healing that had taken place when I gave birth to Beacon, and if I was never able to experience that again, I feared I would live in this shadow forever.

In the midst of my anger, I looked out the window and saw my magnolia. Four of the buds had now blossomed into blooms and two little buds remained the same. That very moment, I felt God speak, and this was His promise to me: "You will have four children on earth, and I'll hold two in heaven until you get here to hold your babies yourself." I felt as if my heart might explode, and only my skin was holding me together. God loved me, and I could feel His presence in my life. I knew right then, no matter what the doctor believed, God would bless us once more with our fourth child. I didn't know how and I didn't know when, but my spirit was immediately calmed. I had faith God would deliver His promise no matter how long that might take.

I have seen his Word fulfilled so many times in my life before that I had no reason to doubt Him. I had always prayed God would show me a sign so clear that I wouldn't be able to miss it. Even though that little tree never grew or bloomed in four years, He allowed it to bud right when I needed it to. I don't think that is by chance, and I don't think anything is too hard for God. It gives me chills today and tears stream down my face as I share His goodness with you.

As the next couple of weeks passed, the four beautiful blooms on the little

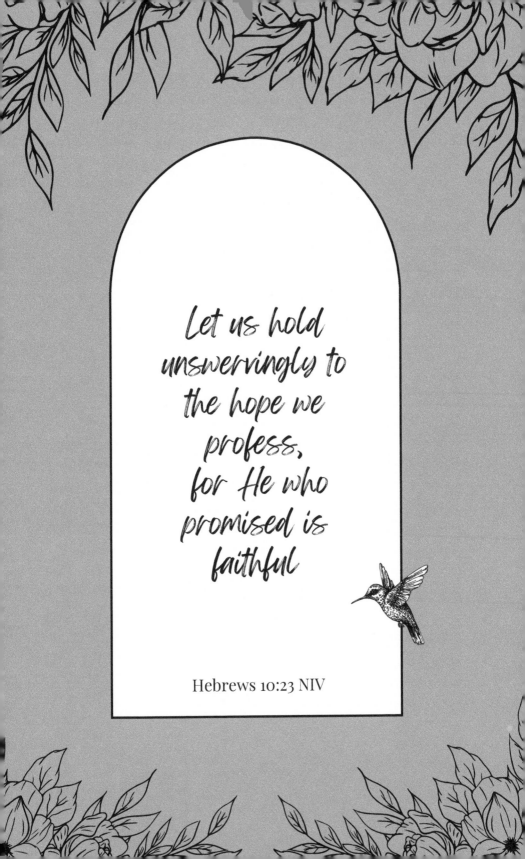

Let us hold unswervingly to the hope we profess, for He who promised is faithful

Hebrews 10:23 NIV

magnolia began to close. The petals fell to the ground, but the two other buds never opened or changed shape. This seemed even more apparent to me that they were a symbol for the babies I had lost. hey remained buds and never bloomed into a flower. Every day while driving by, I was reminded of God's promise and the blessing I hoped would be coming in the future.

Think about how you can relate to this story. Can you think of a moment in your life when you thought there was no hope, no possible way God could change your circumstances? Have you been told by others to give up on your dream or the one thing you have been longing for, for weeks or even years? Friend, I'm here telling you today that whatever you've been fervently praying for, whatever that longing is in your life, nothing is too hard for God. Grow your faith and challenge Him to show up in your life in the type of way that only He could. While you wait, wait in faith. Keep your eyes open, look up from your phone, and take in the masterpiece he is painting in front of you. Don't miss out on this blessing, a remarkable message from God.

"So we're not giving up. How could we! Even though on the outside it often looks like things are falling apart on us, on the inside, where God is making new life, not a day goes by without his unfolding grace. These hard times are small potatoes compared to the coming good times, the lavish celebration prepared for us. There's far more here than meets the eye. The things we see now are here today, gone tomorrow. But the things we can't see now will last forever."
2 Corinthians 4:16-18, MSG

Chapter 14

Unexpected Miracles

> Let us hold unswervingly
> to the hope we profess,
> for He who promised is faithful.
> Hebrews 10:23, NIV

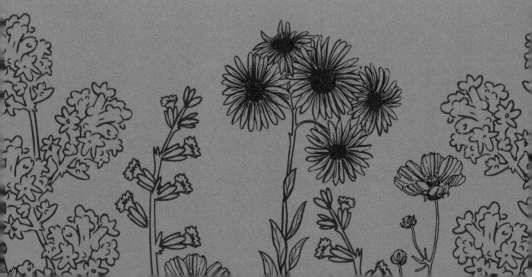

Let us hold unswervingly to the hope we
profess, for He who promised is faithful.
Hebrews 10:23, NIV

A month had passed since the last bloom had fallen from my magnolia tree, and I found myself in an all too familiar position, yet again, sitting in the bathroom holding a pregnancy test in my hands. This time, I was prepared for the answer, no matter what that might be. Like the beautiful verse Hebrews 10:23 says, I had a promise, and I held onto that promise without wavering. Considering I had barely had time to process all of my emotions from the loss and the news from the doctor just a few weeks prior, I didn't expect God to give us another pregnancy this month. I didn't even really know what to expect from my menstrual cycle because, after a miscarriage, your body can do out-of-the-ordinary things — your period could cycle twice in one month or not even come at all for several months thereafter. However, my cheap, bulk box of pregnancy tests had just been delivered, and the test I was holding in my hand slowly revealed two pink lines. I stared in disbelief as the lines got darker and more clear to me. It was a definite positive test. I must document that I have never felt more shocked than at this moment in my life.

I immediately fumbled to gather another test from the box and make sure this was an accurate result because I just wasn't able to wrap my mind around how I could be pregnant and how positive the test in front of me appeared. I watched, through tears, as it became more evident that the second test indeed had two pink lines as well. At that moment, my doubts began to fade, and I knew God had sent His promise, just as He said He would. I wish I could tell you those two tests were all I needed to clear the doubts that consumed my mind, but friends, I guess I'm just not that religious of a person. I'm a doubtful human, and while I'm spilling the truth, I will tell you I ended up taking the entire box of twenty-five tests over the next week (*ahhhh*, embarrassing right?). I even videoed all of the results and sent them to my best friend (who is a nurse) in hopes that her response would reassure the doubts that were consuming my mind, I was really pregnant. I remember her response: "Wow, you take enough tests? I'd say those are definitely positive!" But I just couldn't keep myself from taking more tests. Every time I saw that positive result pop up, I was reassured my baby was in my womb and was safely continuing to grow. I was so grateful to be carrying God's promise and that He had chosen to fulfill this miracle in my life by giving us a baby the doctors said would never be possible to conceive.

A few weeks passed, and it was the Sunday before our first ultrasound. We were getting ready for church while listening to "Fear Is A Liar" by Zach Williams. This song had been on repeat for Brenton and constantly pronounced peace over his spirit through the many trials we had gone through in the past few months. When we got in the car, the same song began playing on the radio as we drove to church. (By chance? I think not). Brenton\ explained, "Every time he needs something in his life, God sends a song as a promise that everything will be okay." I just love when God works like this, don't you? I also love how God speaks to all of us in different ways, unique to our specific needs and personality.

Just as we got settled in the pew at church, Pastor Marty walked onto the stage. He opened his Bible and the scripture he began to read rang a very familiar tune in my ear. He read from Genesis 22.

1After these things God tested Abraham and said to him, "Abraham!" And he said, "Here I am." 2He said, "Take your son, your only son Isaac, whom you love, and go to the land of Moriah, and offer him there as a burnt offering on one of the mountains of which I shall tell you." 3So Abraham rose early in the morning, saddled his donkey, and took two of his young men with him, and his son Isaac. And he cut the wood for the burnt offering and arose and went to the place of which God had told him. 4On the third day Abraham lifted up his eyes and saw the place from afar. 5Then Abraham said to his young men, "Stay here with the donkey; I and the boy will go over there and worship and come again to you." 6And Abraham took the wood of the burnt offering and laid it on Isaac his son. And he took in his hand the fire and the knife. So they went both of them together. 7And Isaac said to his father Abraham, "My father!" And he said, "Here I am, my son." He said, "Behold, the fire and the wood, but where is the lamb for a burnt offering?" 8Abraham said, "God will provide for himself the lamb for a burnt offering, my son." So they went both of them together. 9When they came to the place of which God had told him, Abraham built the altar there and laid the wood in order and bound Isaac his son and laid him on the altar, on top of the wood. 10Then Abraham reached out his hand and took the knife to slaughter his son. 11But the angel of the Lord called to him from heaven and said, "Abraham, Abraham!" And he said, "Here I am." 12He said, "Do not lay your hand on the boy or do anything to him, for now I know that you fear God, seeing you have not withheld your son, your only son, from me." 13And Abraham lifted up his eyes and looked, and behold, behind him was a ram, caught in a thicket by his horns. And Abraham went and took the ram and offered it up as a burnt offering instead of his son. 14So Abraham called the name of that place, "The Lord will provide"; as it is said to this day, "On the mount of the Lord it shall be provided." 15And the angel of the Lord called to Abraham a second time from heaven 16and said, "By myself I have sworn, declares the Lord, because you have done this and have not withheld your son, your only son, 17I will surely bless you, and I will surely multiply your offspring as the stars of heaven and as the sand that is on the seashore. And your offspring shall possess the gate of his enemies, 18and in your offspring shall all the nations of the earth be blessed, because you have obeyed my voice."

Genesis 22:1-18, ESV

While he was reading, I realized this scripture was not about Abraham and Sarah, as I thought it would be, but it was all about Abraham and his son, Isaac. If you're not familiar with this scripture, it's an amazing story of how God instructed Abraham to sacrifice His promised son Isaac on an altar because He had no lamb. Unlike today, back then, you were instructed to sacrifice a spotless animal as an offering to the Lord to cover and pay for the sins. (Thank God we don't have to do this anymore since Jesus paid that price for

After all this, God tested Abraham.
God said, "Abraham!"
"Yes?" answered Abraham. "I'm listening."
He said, "Take your dear son Isaac whom you love and go to the land of Moriah. Sacrifice him there as a burnt offering on one of the mountains that I'll point out to you."
Abraham got up early in the morning and saddled his donkey. He took two of his young servants and his son Isaac. He had split wood for the burnt offering. He set out for the place God had directed him. On the third day he looked up and saw the place in the distance. Abraham told his two young servants, "Stay here with the donkey. The boy and I are going over there to worship; then we'll come back to you."
Abraham took the wood for the burnt offering and gave it to Isaac his son to carry. He carried the flint and the knife. The two of them went off together.
Isaac said to Abraham his father, "Father?"
"Yes, my son."
"We have flint and wood, but where's the sheep for the burnt offering?"
Abraham said, "Son, God will see to it that there's a sheep for the burnt offering." And they kept on walking together.

Genesis 22:1-8, MSG

all of us.) Abraham fully trusted in God, that He would provide a sacrifice, yet out of obedience to God, he climbed the mountain, built an altar, and followed through with everything God had instructed Him to do. In the very last second, God spoke and gave Abraham a sacrifice so he wouldn't have to harm his son whom he had waited for Sarah to conceive for over forty years. God fulfilled His promise, allowing Abraham to raise Isaac and making him known as "the child of promise" throughout history. During this sermon, I couldn't help but laugh and cry at the same time. He spoke not only of Isaac reaping the benefits of God's promises to Abraham and Sarah but also of Isaac's children receiving the blessings and his children's children and so on. To the present day, we are still receiving the blessings and promises of God. I was in complete awe of God's amazingness, and His willingness to speak to me so clearly. I knew, through these scriptures, my ultrasound was going to go well; I knew my baby was going to have a heartbeat. I knew the storm of loss was over, because I had already lived it, and I refused to give up on God. I held tightly to the futuristic promises he sent through the hummingbirds and the magnolias in my life, and now was the time to live in it.

Most people don't think God is still working like this in people's lives today, but dear friends, He is. He really is! You just have to open your eyes to see it and open your heart to experience it. He is all-powerful and is still performing great miracles today. Just as He has spoken these words to me time and again, He wants to speak to you. One of my fears in writing this book was to sound repetitive because God has used some of the same things to speak to me throughout my life over and over again, but that's our "thing." I want to tell you all of these details, not so you will now pay attention every time you hear the words Abraham and Sarah or every time you pass by a magnolia tree, but to open your eyes to your "thing," your communication with God. Pay attention to the things in your path that God might be using to speak to you directly every single day. Open your eyes to the answer He's sending to the questions you have been asking Him that are right in front of your face.

Over the next few weeks, I had issues with spotting and a few scares that a traumatized mama never wants to go through, yet every time thereafter, the

Mary has been the most influential "Mother" there ever was, and yet her journey was extremely difficult, it was hard and full of obstacles. She overcame each one of those strenuous moments through her faith and complete dependence on God, and infinite trust that His plan was necessary.

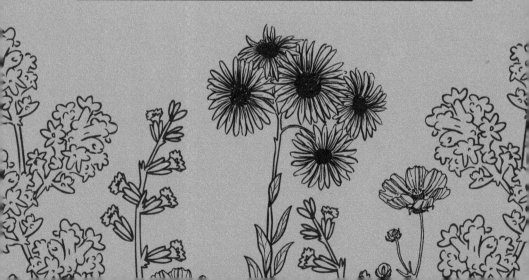

bloodwork and ultrasounds showed that our little peanut was a fighter and was doing completely fine. We found out we were having another little girl, and I continually felt like she was already so brave. She was my little fighter that beat all of the odds and, from the very beginning, was determined to call me mama. We decided to name her Braven Wilder to honor the strength she was given even at conception. Now, I wish I could tell you how wonderful this pregnancy progressed. I also wish I could tell you how magical the delivery went. I even wish I could tell you how, once she arrived, we had no issues at all, but unfortunately, I can't tell you any of that. This pregnancy was honestly the absolute worst of all of my other pregnancies combined. I was considered high risk with stroke-level blood pressure, and unlike the pregnancies with my others, I was in the doctor's office twice a week to monitor my body and check on our baby girl. I felt like I spent more time worrying I would lose her. It was a hard year full of ups and downs and, quite frankly, the opposite of what I imagined the birth of a promised child to be. Throughout this grueling year, my faith was put to the test like never before, and I held tightly to the promise God had given me, and thereafter, His promise indeed remained true. I delivered Braven three weeks early, and although we went through a lot of extremely scary moments once she was here concerning both of our health, we made it, and God's promise was fulfilled.

Looking back on my difficult pregnancy and especially my delivery with Braven, I am reminded of Mary. Now, before you cast judgmental eyes, please know I don't equalize the promise God gave to me with the promise He gave to Mary, a virgin who carried and delivered Jesus, the Christ child. However, when I look at all that Mary had to endure during her pregnancy and especially during her delivery in that barn, I feel a connection with her, and this is why. Jesus' birth is the most important birth of all time, we know this. An angel directly delivered the promise of Mary's miraculous pregnancy to her, telling her she would carry the Messiah for nine months in her womb and that He would thereafter carry the weight of the entire world and the future of every human on His shoulders to save us all from Hell. Can you imagine the burden of that promise Mary must have felt? Can you envision the stress she was under while she was pregnant, knowing it was her sole responsibility to safely carry Jesus in her womb and deliver Him into this imperfect world without a flaw? The conditions were so much worse in those days, yet she had to keep her body protected and healthy during her entire pregnancy. They didn't have fancy doctor's offices, delivery rooms, prenatal vitamins, maternity leggings, and if you need one more, they definitely didn't have the extra large menstrual pads we refer to as diapers and must wear after delivery (Yikes, and who would think those were luxury items?). This changes our perspective on Mary a little, am I right? So many things we think are common, non-luxurious items were not even available to Mary "Jesus' mother" in the slightest. She too endured a difficult journey, yet she was given the most important task no other woman has ever been given in history. Can you relate to her trials at all yet? I think sometimes in life when things get tough, we think God has abandoned us in our time of need, but that's not what He has done at all. God is always right here with us. He is unfailing, and sometimes the precise outcome God has designed for our lives requires a difficult journey.

Mary has been the most influential "mother" there ever was, and yet, her journey was extremely difficult. It was hard and full of obstacles. She overcame each one of those strenuous moments through her faith, complete dependence on God, and infinite trust that His plan was necessary. Oh, how I wish I could go back in time, talk with her, give her a long hug, and tell her how nothing she ever did went unnoticed. I am so thankful for her *yes* that day, which led to my salvation when I was five years old. Mary's trust in God led to the salvation of the entire world, and her unshakable faith in HIS promise gave me strength to trust Him again with the promises He had given to me. You too can have a Mary-type faith and trust in God with the battle He has placed into your hands. All you have to do is be willing to say yes to the journey ahead, no matter how difficult it may be. There is purpose in it, I promise.

And he came to her and said,
"Greetings, O favored one, the Lord is with you!"
But she was greatly troubled at the saying,
and tried to discern what sort
of greeting this might be. And the angel said to her,
"Do not be afraid, Mary,
for you have found favor with God. And behold,
you will conceive in your womb and bear a son,
and you shall call his name Jesus. He will be great and
will be called the Son of the Most High. And the Lord
God will give to Him the throne of His Father David,
and He will reign over the house of David,
and of His kingdom there will be no end."
And Mary said to the angel,
"How will this be since I am a virgin?"
And the angel answered her,
"The Holy Spirit will come upon you,
and the power of the Most High will overshadow you;
therefore the child to be born will be called
holy- the Son of God.

Luke 1:28-35, ESV

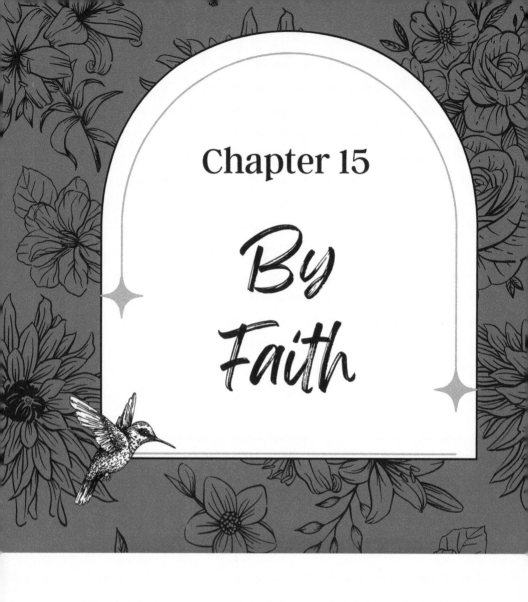

Chapter 15

By Faith

And it is impossible to please God without faith. Anyone who wants to come to Him must believe that God exists and that He rewards those who sincerely seek Him.

Hebrews 11:6, NLT

*The fundamental fact of existence is that this trust in God, this faith,
is the firm foundation under everything that makes life worth
living. It's our handle on what we can't see. The act of faith is what
distinguished our ancestors, set them above the crowd.*
Hebrews 11:6, NLT

Before experiencing my first miscarriage, hummingbirds congregated on the front porch of my home every single day. From early spring to late autumn, many of those beautiful birds fluttered through my flower beds and continuously peeked into my living room through the large picture window on the front of my farmhouse. I had always felt so connected to them, and through that connection, God revealed Himself and His plans for my life many times, as I have shared with you earlier in this book. On the day I endured my first miscarriage, I prayed He would no longer use hummingbirds to communicate with me relating to pregnancy in any way, shape, or form. My outlook on them had been completely changed from that day forward, and my faith in their symbol for my life was shaken. What once had brought such joy and promise to my situation now reminded me of what was ripped from me and the agonizing pain I endured along the way. That hummingbird was, in fact, the last one I had seen on my property for several years after that very day. There were no longer tiny flutters on my porch, little eyes peering in my windows, or any hummingbirds crossing my path as I walked through our backyard. Not a single hummingbird was in sight. God honored my prayer that day by removing them from my life for a period of time which I needed to heal. This is literally a miracle in itself because hummingbirds truly have great memories, and no matter how far they migrate throughout the winter months, they typically always return to the same yards, flowers, and feeders year after year. I had always been a lover of hummingbirds since I was a child, and I learned all sorts of interesting facts about birds from my Nanny. When I was little,

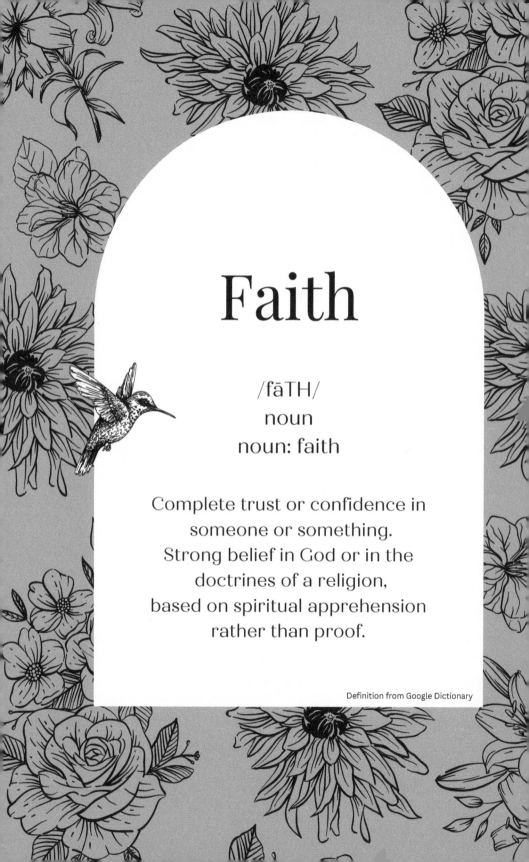

Faith

/fāTH/
noun
noun: faith

Complete trust or confidence in
someone or something.
Strong belief in God or in the
doctrines of a religion,
based on spiritual apprehension
rather than proof.

Definition from Google Dictionary

she taught me the importance of planting specific flowers in our yard to bring in coordinating species of birds. Thanks to her lessons, my flower beds are full of well-established hydrangeas, hosta, gardenias, and verbena, all of which hummingbirds love, so considering the fact that I refrained from hanging the hummingbird feeder for a few seasons wouldn't have affected whether they would come back to my house or not.

After a few years of absence, I remember the first hummingbird to make its appearance at our house. It was the week I delivered Braven, our last child, and the only thing on my to-do list right after having a c-section was to sit in my favorite comfy spot on the couch while snuggling my sweet newborn baby (and binge-watching Hallmark movies, but that's beside the fact). This specific spot I sat in daily had the most perfect view of the front yard, which is one of the reasons I always chose to sit there. One day, while I sat there cuddling and taking in the sweet aroma of my newborn baby, I caught a glimpse of a tiny little bird wisping by my window. I sat completely still as the little bird flew back and forth like it was searching for something until it softly landed on the string lights hanging across my front porch. The spot it perched on has a direct view into my living room, and in years prior, was a regular hang-out spot for all of the hummingbirds. I didn't move as we appeared to be playing a round of the starring game. As we both remained still taking in each other's appearances, my emotions began to take over, and I began to cry. I was holding God's promise in my arms, and I felt this little bird was a message sent to me from God to remind me that my infertility journey was over. It was a miracle in itself that God returned the hummingbirds back to my farm at the most uncommon time, the end of summer since that's usually when they begin migrating south. Also, this was His perfect timing, revealing it to me at the very moment my last baby was safely nestled in my arms. This all made it evident this was a message straight from the Holy Spirit that I would never encounter loss or fertility issues again (PRAISE JESUS!). I felt a freedom that day I hadn't felt in twelve years as I reflected on all that I had encountered in my life leading up to this moment. I was free from it all, and this little bird was sent as a promise that it was finished. Oh my, what a powerful moment in my life this was, and I'll never get over it. Since that day, hummingbirds continually gather around our farmhouse from early April to late September, and the significance they once held in my life has now been restored. I rarely step outside without one circling around me, confirming its presence and purpose in my life. They're such a beautiful reminder of everything God has ever spoken to me and delivered in His perfect timing. He wants to do these same things for you as well.

The fundamental fact of existence is that this trust in God, this faith,
is the firm foundation under everything that makes life worth living.
It's our handle on what we can't see. The act of faith is what
distinguished our ancestors, set them above the crowd.
Hebrews 11:1-2, MSG

I LOVE this scripture in Hebrews. It speaks so profoundly. As I walked this journey, I questioned God time and time again. *Why? Why did I have to face difficulties along the way? Why did I have to go through loss? Why did I have to wait to conceive each of my children? Why did He choose me for this specific path? And why did He speak to me so clearly throughout my life in ways so detailed it's hard for other people to understand?* The answer has been so clouded and unclear for me until I read these words tonight. I must admit to you I am a bit shaken as I have had these unanswered questions on repeat in my mind for a long time, and God just revealed the answer for me, and it is this: God's plan for me today, ultimately determines the result of my tomorrow and every day thereafter. This means everything we go through in life, whether we view it as good or bad, determines the precise result of our future and our children's future and even their children's future. Ultimately, God is the only one that can see the purpose those choices have on our tomorrow. As we learn this, it's more important than ever to grow our faith in God and trust that by faith, all things through Christ are attainable. We must trust God, even when He delivers the hardest path and the most excruciating circumstances. He knows what is ultimately best for our lives.

By faith we understand that the entire universe was formed
at God's command, that what we now see did not

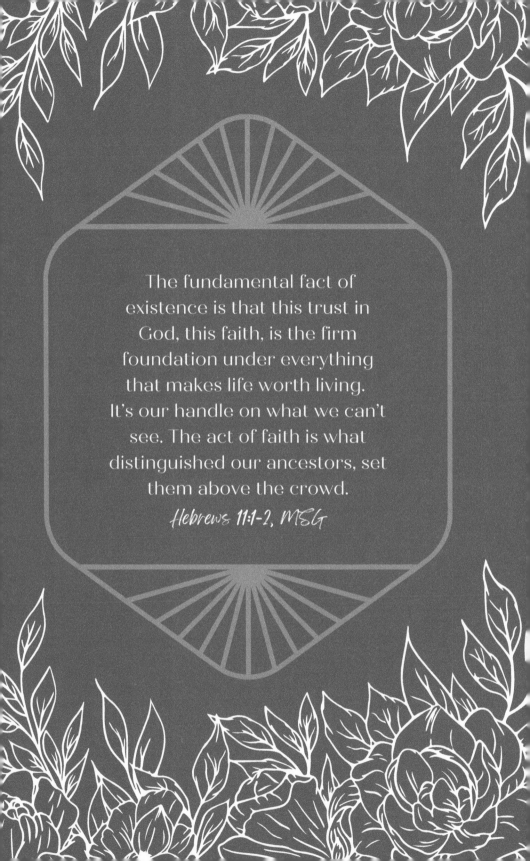

The fundamental fact of
existence is that this trust in
God, this faith, is the firm
foundation under everything
that makes life worth living.
It's our handle on what we can't
see. The act of faith is what
distinguished our ancestors, set
them above the crowd.

Hebrews 11:1-2, MSG

come from anything that can be seen.
Hebrews 11:3, NLT

"By faith ... " Now, I have heard sermons on this before, and I have never quite wrapped my mind around the meaning of it because faith, to me, just meant believing in the existence of God and trusting He sent His Son Jesus to save us from our sins when He died on the cross. I had never questioned this fact and had faith in these truths since I was a small child. I recall many conversations with people throughout the past few years, telling them of the miraculous moments God had placed in my life, and the response I heard the most was, "Wow, what a huge faith you have!" Upon hearing this, I have always paused not knowing how to respond because, truthfully, throughout this journey, I had never seen what I have been through having anything to do with "my" faith but having everything to do with the presence of The Almighty God in my life. This still remains true, but, as I read this scripture, it's telling us that the FAITH we have in The Almighty God to do the very things He has promised in His Word does, in fact, hold significance.

The Bible says:

> *It was by faith that even Sarah was able to have a*
> *child, Though she was barren and was too old. She*
> *believed that God would keep His promise.*
> Hebrews 11:11, NLT

This scripture confirms that it was by faith Sarah was able to conceive. This is telling us there is importance in the faith that she had. She believed in the promise God gave to her. She had faith and believed in Him, even after wanting a child for over seventy years. As I searched back, I found it appears Sarah married Abraham around the age of forty-five. In that day, the main reason to wed someone would be to reproduce, since the population of mankind was very slim. This tells us she was hoping to become pregnant for about forty years when God told her she would have a son. Can you imagine waiting forty years for anything? Wow, this makes my two to five-year wait seem so small in comparison to hers, yet in my opinion, her faith remained incredibly strong as she clung to the word God had delivered to her. I want to have faith like Sarah, don't you?

The Bible says:

> *And so a whole nation came from this one man who was as good as dead - a nation with so many people that, like the stars in the sky and the sand on the seashore, there is no way to count them.*
> Hebrews 11:12, NLT

Can I just say *WOW*! Do you see what this means? "And so a whole nation came from this man who was as good as dead..." What a miracle in itself. From one man and woman who had passed the age of childbearing, was brought forth an abundance of life. So not only does Sarah's faith in God and the promise He gave to her affect her happiness and privilege of finally becoming a mother, but it also affects the generations and generations of people who, through the lineage, eventually bring us to our existence on this earth. All of this by God's mighty hand and undying faith in Him. Looking at this scripture, I'm brought back to each of the big moments in my life. Until now, I never realized how much God deeply honors an unshakable faith in Him, and I honestly never want to doubt Him or His plans ever again. God's timing is perfect, and He will always keep His word. If He says it, it will be done. Don't doubt Him and never lose faith.

In the same chapter in Hebrews, we see how every one of these big moments listed here in the scriptures where miracles were performed, was all done by faith. Verse 7 speaks of Noah saying, " ... and by faith [he] built the ark believing the flood was coming." Verse 30 says, "By faith the people of Israel marched around Jericho, and the walls came crashing down" (NLT). Are you seeing the trend here yet? My favorite, though, is towards the end when it says,

> *How much more do I need to say? It would take too long to recount the stories of Gideon, Barak, Samson, Jephthah, David, Samuel, and*

"God's plan for your today, ultimately determines the results of your tomorrow and everyday thereafter."

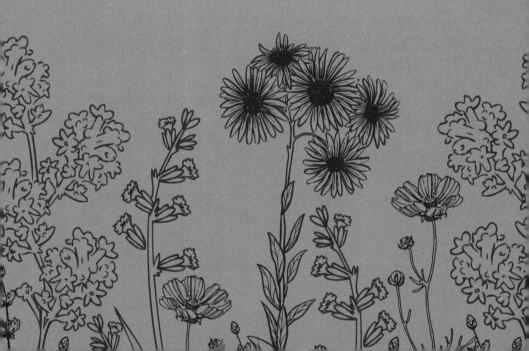

all the prophets. By faith these people overthrew kingdoms, ruled
with justice, and received what God had promised them. They shut
the mouths of lions, quenched the flames of fire, and escaped
death by the edge of the sword. Their weakness was turned to strength.
They became strong in battle And put whole armies to flight.
Hebrews 11:32-34, ESV

Can you imagine if this verse had continued on, how long it would be? I would love to think eventually it would get to me. I would love to think eventually it would get to you as well. How strong is your faith today? Are you trusting in the word God has given you? Or, do you continually question Him and ask for more confirmations? Hold fast today to the promise and word from God you have received and guard your heart against the doubtful influences and non-believers of this world. Cling to this instruction God has given to us:

"Truly I tell you, if you have faith as small as a mustard seed,
you can say to this mountain, 'Move from here to there', and it
will move. Nothing will be impossible for you."
Matthew 17:20, ESV

Now, I want to take a moment to mention, we must be careful not to misinterpret these scriptures while planning out our own will and path for our lives. In fact, my pastor recently said this scripture in Matthew 17 is one of the most misquoted and taken out-of-context scriptures. So, the lesson we should gather from this scripture isn't that we can do all things by faith. No. The ultimate lesson here is realizing how much value God places on our faith in Him. He wants us to believe when He says it, it will be done, even if it takes Him 20 years to carry out His ultimate plan.

These verses on faith are not instructing us to profess our own goals and dreams by proclaiming "that by faith," anything and everything we prophesy for our own lives will be possible. For instance, tomorrow, I will not wake up and set an unattainable goal of becoming a world champion arm wrestler by faith in Jesus Christ. Now, I have mentioned before I inherited these big 'ole arms from my Nanny, but I completely understand God isn't going to suddenly put them to good use in a magical way just because I profess limitless faith in Him to do so. What I am talking about, though, is having *unconditional faith* in the plan God has ultimately laid before you. If He has given you a sequence for your life, He will prevail. His journey might take longer than you hoped, but keep the faith, knowing HE will do as He has said He will.

> *Some faced jeers and flogging, and even chains and imprisonment.*
> *They were put to death by stoning; they were sawed in two; they were*
> *killed by the sword. They went about in sheepskins and goatskins,*
> *destitute, persecuted and mistreated— the world was not worthy*
> *of them. They wandered in deserts and mountains, living in*
> *caves and in holes in the ground. These were all commended for*
> *their faith, yet none of them received what had been promised,*
> *since God had planned something better for us so that only*
> *together with us would they be made perfect.*
> Hebrews 11:36-40, NIV

This scripture is hard to read, but oh so important to acknowledge. We see here the Bible mentions notable people who devoted their lives to God, yet in the end, they suffered immensely or died a cruel death for Jesus' namesake. This would appear, to us, their prayers went completely unanswered and that the unfailing faith they had went unnoticed by God, but this is not true at all. It is saying here He had something much better in His plans for them; plans to gain a glorious life in Heaven, living in perfection with God through eternity. As it says in Philippians 1:21 (NLT): "For to me, living means living for Christ, and dying is even better." We, too, have the assurance to die is to gain a whole new everlasting life with God in Heaven, by faith, through Jesus Christ. He is truly the ultimate reward.

Think for a moment about those instances in your life in which you wholeheartedly believed God was going to intervene in a certain way, yet your specific prayer went unanswered. For you, this might bring to mind a loved one you thought would survive, but in the end, didn't make it through, or a rela-

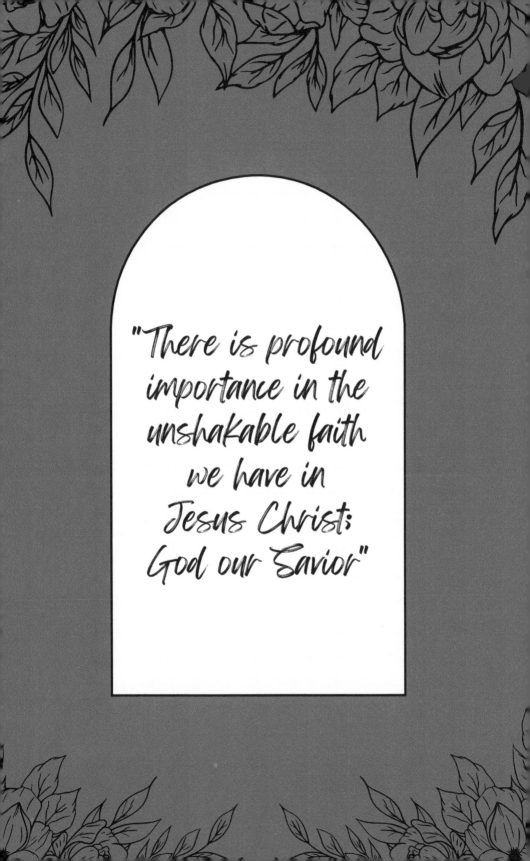

"There is profound importance in the unshakable faith we have in Jesus Christ; God our Savior"

tionship you hoped wouldn't come to an end. Or, perhaps something else perhaps comes to mind when you reflect on a prayer you wholly believed and had complete faith God would intervene in, yet, it had an altogether different outcome than you ever imagined. This might have made you feel as if God had deserted you and didn't love you by honoring your faith in Him. But, what if our request altered the life of another, preventing them from the moment they got to see the face of Jesus? What if we hindered them from obtaining a life of everlasting perfection, all so we could hold them here on this earth a little while longer? I personally don't think they would like us to be in charge of plans like that, do you?

Rest in knowing this fact: God honors an unshakable faith in Him. He adores complete trust in the Word He has already given. We understand as Christians He doesn't "need" our faith in Him to perform anything. He is God, and He CAN do anything He wants, at any given moment in time, with or without our faith in Him. However, these scriptures utterly convey there is profound importance in the unshakable faith we have in Jesus Christ, God our Savior. God is and will always be GOD, no matter how unstable our faith becomes. He has placed a significant value on the faith we have in Him, and I want to be willing to trust Him, no matter what the ultimate outcome is for my life. God has my BEST waiting for me and you as well. So friend, when you are angry, keep the faith. When you are hurting, keep the faith. When you are consumed by doubt, keep the faith. Trust God is in control, unconditionally loves us, and has our best outcome in His ultimate plan.

Faith
Complete trust or confidence in someone or something.
Strong belief in God or in the doctrines of a religion,
based on spiritual apprehension rather than proof.[8]

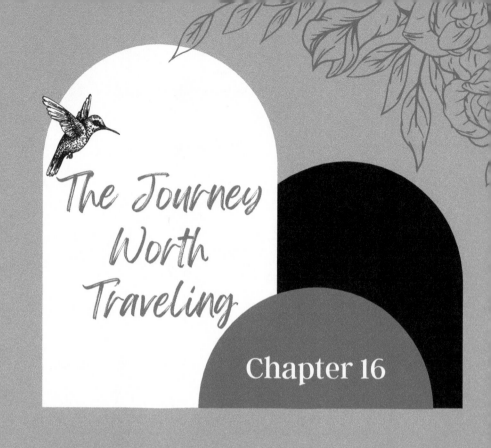

The Journey Worth Traveling

Chapter 16

"God never said that the journey
would be easy,
But He did say that the arrival
would be worthwhile."
-Max Lucado

"God never said that the journey would be easy, But He did say that the arrival would be worthwhile."
Max Lucado, pastor, speaker, and best-selling author[9]

The journey to and through motherhood did not come easily for me, but it has been completely worth it. I can honestly say if I had the chance to go back to the very beginning and I could choose one of two paths laid before me, one being no miscarriages, no years of trying for babies and infertility struggles, and the other with four quick pregnancies, four healthy babies, simple, easy, and done, I would absolutely choose the long, hard path over and over again. Why you might ask? The answers to that question, for me, are:

The heart of man plans his way,
but the LORD establishes his steps.
Proverbs 16:9, ESV

1. The journey you take changes the result of your life and, ultimately, the person you become. I'll explain. For me, had my journey been easy, I would be a completely different type of mother to my children. I wouldn't fully appreciate how individually special they are had I have never been told I wouldn't be able to conceive them. I would never have prayed over each one of them in the way I did when I longed so deeply for them to be in my womb, and my heart wouldn't have had the chance to languish for them for the years at a time I did. This made the fulfillment of motherhood so much more amazing once it was given. If you erased the two miscarriages I endured from existence, you would be eliminating many painful memories, longings, and agonizing moments from my life. But, in taking away that pain, it would also completely take away my babies. This would mean eliminating two little babies I loved, longed for, and labored into Heaven, and this is something I will never be okay with. As

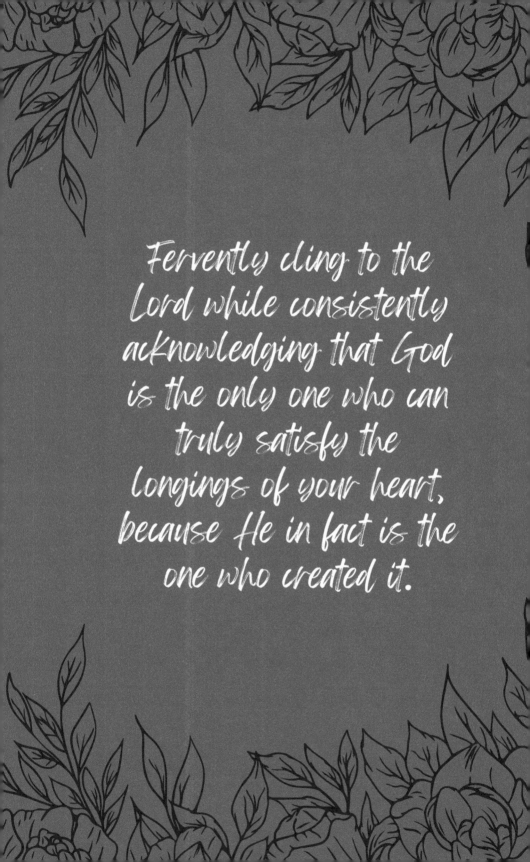

Fervently cling to the Lord while consistently acknowledging that God is the only one who can truly satisfy the longings of your heart, because He in fact is the one who created it.

the saying goes, "Better to have loved and lost than never to have loved at all."[10] This is true for me in terms of miscarriage. I was their momma on earth for a short time while I carried each one in my womb, but in Heaven, I will have everlasting life with both of them. Knowing this fact makes every trial worth it. When I enter Heaven's gates and run to my babies, *OH* what a day of rejoicing that will be as I get to hold my little ones for the very first time. On this day, I will finally be identified as who I truly am inside, "a Momma of SIX children".

Don't copy the behavior and customs of this world,
But let God transform you into a new person by changing
the way you think. Then you will learn to know God's will
for you, which is good and pleasing and perfect.
Romans 12:2 NLT

2. The journey cultivated a lasting connection. My personal relationship with God wouldn't be as significant, because every one of those miraculous moments that took place in my life when I was desperate for a child would never have happened. Nothing in life has ever made me feel more helpless and desperate than in times of longing for motherhood, and God was the only one capable of delivering me from the darkness that consumed my soul during those moments. I am eternally grateful to Him for those significant bits in my life and the pruning of my soul. I'm thankful for the messages He sent through His wondrous creations, growing my faith like never before.

Exalt in His Holy name; rejoice, you who worship the Lord.
Search for the Lord and for His strength; continually seek him.
Remember the wonders He has performed, His miracles and the
rulings He Has given, you children of "Israel" (Isaac) you
descendants of Jacob, his chosen ones.
1 Chronicles 16:10-13, NLT

This brings me to number 3: An undeniable FAITH is obtained by encountering the magnificent works of God. The sentimental value of these words is something I will never EVER get over. As I have written of how my faith has

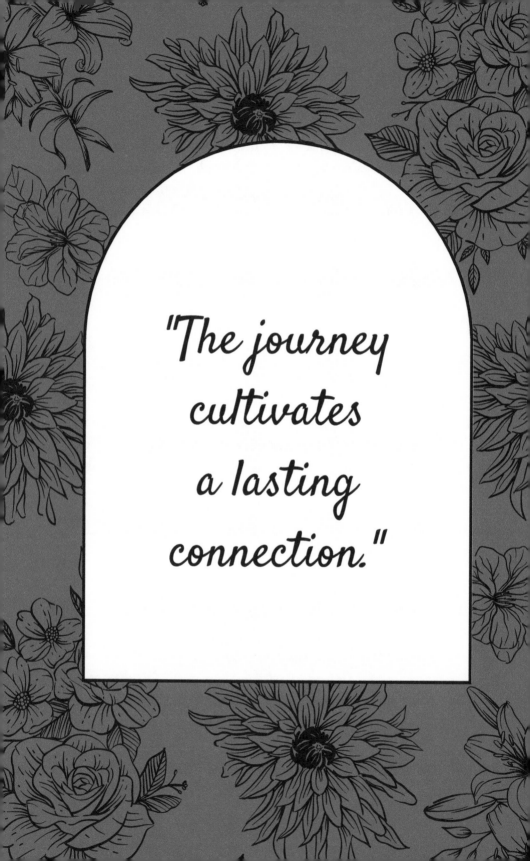

"The journey cultivates a lasting connection."

been put to the test throughout the pages of this book, I now know the unseen growth that took place in the waiting periods was essential to my future. Seeing Him place specific promises on my life, then perfectly deliver them as he told me He would, created an undeniable faith I never thought was possible. I'll never have the same way of thinking again. The Bible tells us faith the size of a mustard seed can move mountains, so what could we move if our faith grew even more than that? I don't want to miss out on a single thing or place He has for my future by living in doubt. I never want to be uncertain of the splendorous presence and power of THE Lord God Almighty.

And it is impossible to please God without faith.
Anyone who wants to come to Him must believe that God
exist and that He rewards those who sincerely seek Him.
Hebrews 11:6, NLT

And lastly, number 4: Had I not had the extra time to cover each longing for pregnancy in prayer, my children's demeanor would be different. I can see how the personalities of each of my children reflect the battle I encountered to get them here. It's so intriguing for me to witness how intricate God's plans are, and though you might question this theory, for me, this has proven true. When I watch each of my children, I see my firstborn, Bentley Mac. He is so particular. He's my little, OCD, Mama pleaser. He loves me with all of his heart. He never wants to upset me or his dad and strives daily to please God in all he does.

My second born, Baize Willow, has a carefree spirit like none of the others. I don't think it's by chance she was conceived faster than all of them and I had the healthiest pregnancy as well. In fact, I don't think my pinky toe even swelled while she was in my belly; it was an extremely easy pregnancy. She, by far, has the strongest personality of all of my children. Nothing breaks her will, and though I didn't work hard to get her here, she makes me work double-time, taming my patience every day of the year. I know she will do great things in this world, and her strength will be magnified to stand firm in her faith and love of the Lord.

My third is my little rainbow baby, Beacon Meadow. This girl is the most well-known of all of my kids because she never meets a stranger. The love of the Lord radiates from her inner soul, and she paints a smile on the face of every person she meets. I have never met a more funny child in my life, and the light she shines on this world is so bright.

This brings me to my last child, Braven Wilder. This little babe is the sweetest and will surely be melting my heart for years and years to come. She has every one of my kids wrapped around her finger, and she is the blessing we prayed for every night at the dinner table. I think she has been prayed over more than any of the other children because they all had a part in longing for and praying over her daily. She's the definition of her name already, and just as we celebrated her first birthday, she was already climbing out of her crib and onto anything she can reach her leg up to. Help us, Lord, with this brave little girl.

Trust in the Lord with all your heart;
Do not depend on your own understanding.
Proverbs 3:5, NLT

Can you see the value of trials yet? I'm telling you all of these things so you will see the importance of God's distinct plans over your own perfectly hand-written path for your life. More often than not, we get impatient as we don't understand. We get angry at God for the way He does things and the time He takes to perfect our journey. But, you must know He is taking the time to make it just that ... PERFECT. The journey you're on was painted only for you to walk on. This means, no one else will have a story just like yours. Nobody else will face the exact trials you might endure. It's your journey. This might sound absolutely terrible when you look at how high some of the bumps in the road might be, but sweet friend, if you just keep pressing through, the destination at the end of that strenuous road will be worth it. The new version of yourself when you reach your destination will be stronger than ever fathomed, with Him by your side, and the relationship you create with God along the way will be magnified. Don't give up now. You may only be a few steps from the one thing you've been longing for. You could be a day away from the mo-

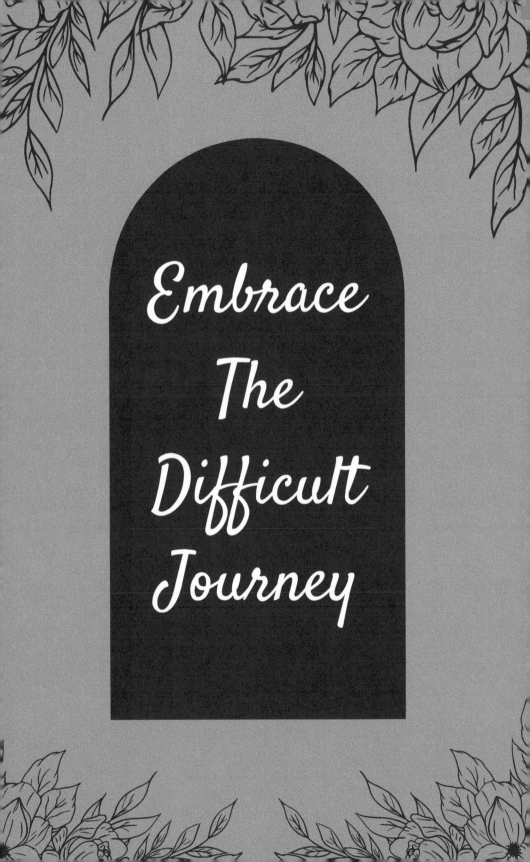

ment you have fervently been praying for, so do not tap out and throw in the towel just yet. You can persevere because God gives us tremendous strength to keep pressing on. You are not alone on this journey; His presence of peace is with you wherever the journey takes you.

You will keep in perfect peace those whose minds are steadfast,
because they trust in you, Trust in the LORD forever,
for the LORD himself, is the Rock eternal.
Isaiah 26:3 & 4, NIV

As you venture through life's rugged journey, there will be longings that captivate your heart and immense desires which briefly consume your mind. In moments like these, when your faith becomes weak, remember this truth: Fervently cling to the Lord while consistently acknowledging God is the only one who can truly satisfy the longings of your heart because He, in fact, is the one who created it.

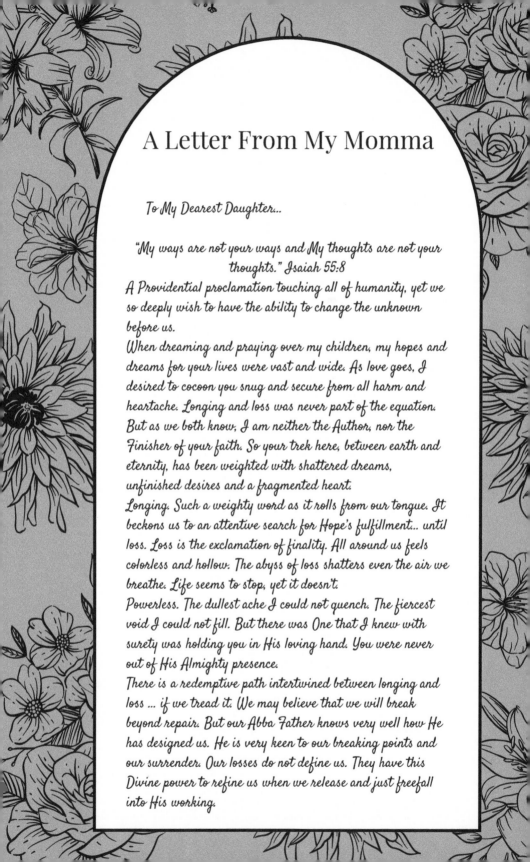

A Letter From My Momma

To My Dearest Daughter...

"My ways are not your ways and My thoughts are not your thoughts." Isaiah 55:8

A Providential proclamation touching all of humanity, yet we so deeply wish to have the ability to change the unknown before us.

When dreaming and praying over my children, my hopes and dreams for your lives were vast and wide. As love goes, I desired to cocoon you snug and secure from all harm and heartache. Longing and loss was never part of the equation. But as we both know, I am neither the Author, nor the Finisher of your faith. So your trek here, between earth and eternity, has been weighted with shattered dreams, unfinished desires and a fragmented heart.

Longing. Such a weighty word as it rolls from our tongue. It beckons us to an attentive search for Hope's fulfillment... until loss. Loss is the exclamation of finality. All around us feels colorless and hollow. The abyss of loss shatters even the air we breathe. Life seems to stop, yet it doesn't.

Powerless. The dullest ache I could not quench. The fiercest void I could not fill. But there was One that I knew with surety was holding you in His loving hand. You were never out of His Almighty presence.

There is a redemptive path intertwined between longing and loss ... if we tread it. We may believe that we will break beyond repair. But our Abba Father knows very well how He has designed us. He is very keen to our breaking points and our surrender. Our losses do not define us. They have this Divine power to refine us when we release and just freefall into His working.

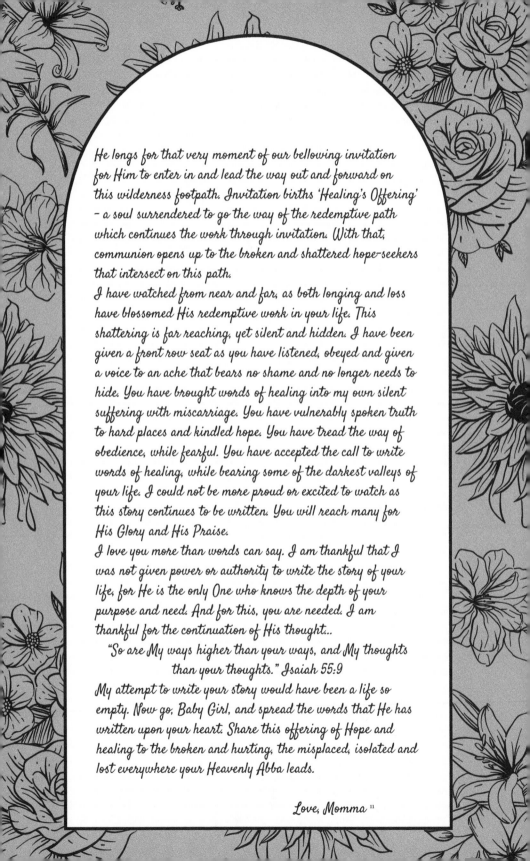

He longs for that very moment of our bellowing invitation for Him to enter in and lead the way out and forward on this wilderness footpath. Invitation births 'Healing's Offering' – a soul surrendered to go the way of the redemptive path which continues the work through invitation. With that, communion opens up to the broken and shattered hope-seekers that intersect on this path.

I have watched from near and far, as both longing and loss have blossomed His redemptive work in your life. This shattering is far reaching, yet silent and hidden. I have been given a front row seat as you have listened, obeyed and given a voice to an ache that bears no shame and no longer needs to hide. You have brought words of healing into my own silent suffering with miscarriage. You have vulnerably spoken truth to hard places and kindled hope. You have tread the way of obedience, while fearful. You have accepted the call to write words of healing, while bearing some of the darkest valleys of your life. I could not be more proud or excited to watch as this story continues to be written. You will reach many for His Glory and His Praise.

I love you more than words can say. I am thankful that I was not given power or authority to write the story of your life, for He is the only One who knows the depth of your purpose and need. And for this, you are needed. I am thankful for the continuation of His thought...

"So are My ways higher than your ways, and My thoughts than your thoughts." Isaiah 55:9

My attempt to write your story would have been a life so empty. Now go, Baby Girl, and spread the words that He has written upon your heart. Share this offering of Hope and healing to the broken and hurting, the misplaced, isolated and lost everywhere your Heavenly Abba leads.

Love, Momma

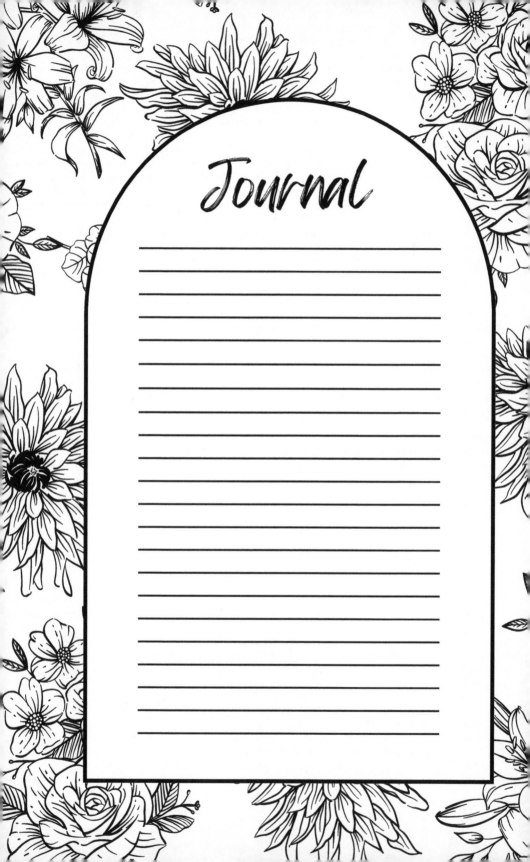

Journal

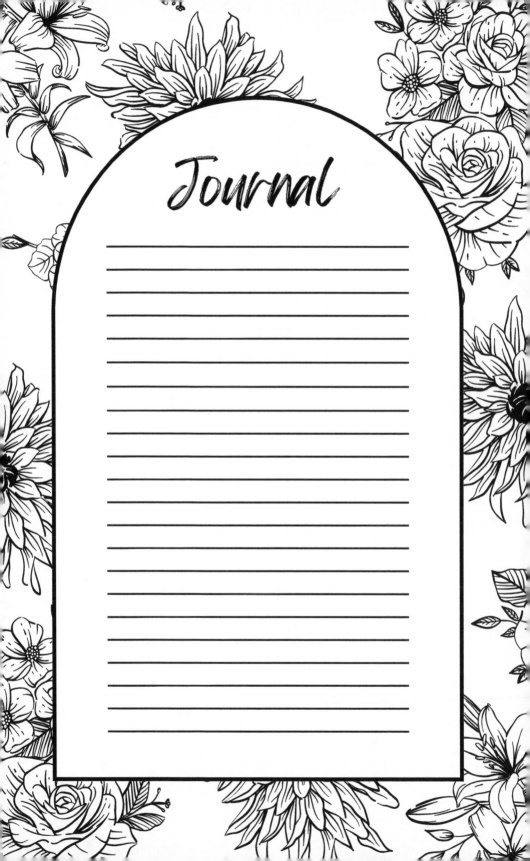

Journal

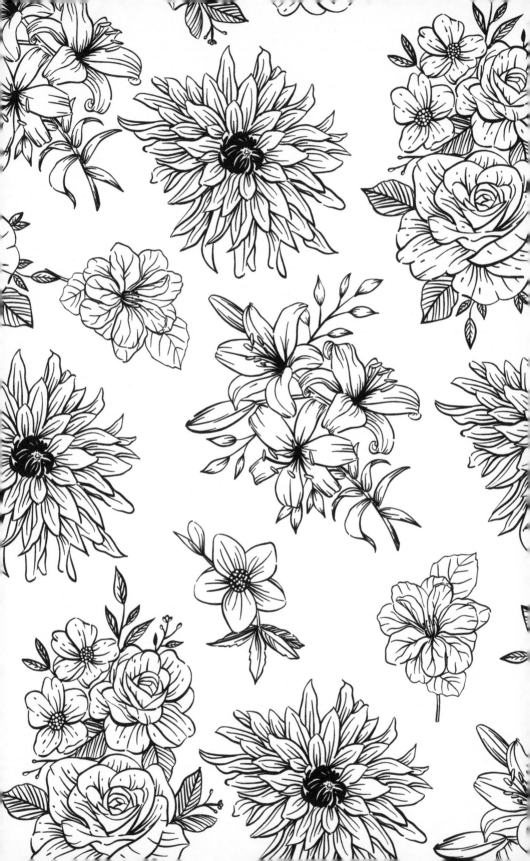

Thank you to my husband for going the extra mile this past year so I could pen down the longings of my heart and the word that God was giving me. Writing a book is no easy task, and you remained kind in the moments my mood reflected the load I was under.

Thank you to United House Publishing for believing in my vision for this book. For the late night calls and support. I'm forever grateful for your encouragement through my struggles.

Thank you to Hannah for managing the coffee shop, being my biggest fan, supporter and always proof reading everything I was unsure of. You're the kindest soul I know.

To my Momma, for this endearing letter I thank you. The world needs a mommas' words like these when their heart is broken. Thank you for encouraging me when I was in doubt, believing in me when I was broken, and complimenting me when I was down on myself.

To my friends, your support means the world to me. I value your kind words, encouragement and direction for my life. I love you all so very much and wouldn't want to go through life without you by my side.

xoxo, Torrie

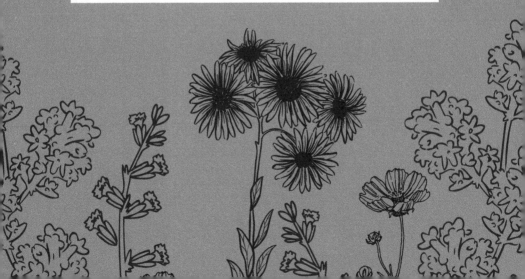

Notes

1. Barton, Dawn. *Laughing Through The Ugly Cry and Funding Unstoppable Joy*. Nashville, TN: Thomas Nelson, 2020.

2. Truity. "The Enneagram Personality Test." truity.com, accessed January 21, 2023, https://www.truity.com/test/enneagram-personality-test.

3. Merriam-Webster.com, s.v. "longing," accessed January 21, 2023, https://www.merriam-webster.com/.

4. Wooten, Linda. A Mother's Thoughts. Amazon, 46, 2014. Kindle.

5. Romans 8:28, NLT

6. Quenby, Siobhan et al. "Miscarriage matters: the epidemiological, physical, psychological, and economic costs of early pregnancy loss." Lancet (London, England) vol. 397,10285 (2021): 1658-1667. doi:10.1016/S0140-6736(21)00682-6.

7. Google dictionary, ed, s.v. "rainbow baby," accessed February 15, 2023, https://www.google.com/search?q=definition+rainbow+baby&source.

8. Google dictionary, ed, s.v. "faith," accessed February 15, 2023, https://www.google.com/search?q=faith&source.

9. Lucado, Max. *Let the Journey Begin: Finding God's Best for Your Life*. Nashville: Thomas Nelson, 2015.

10. Tennyson, Lord Alfred. In Memoriam A.H.H., 1833.

11. Letter from Torrie's Mother-Sharon Bollinger, Author for Proverbs 31, Speaker & Pastor's Wife.

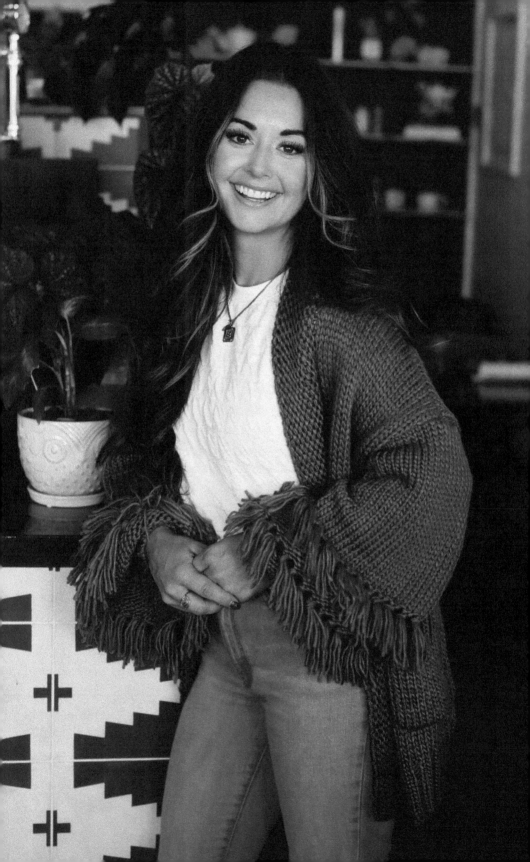

About the Author

Torrie Jarrett is the co-owner and founder of Willowbrook Enterprises. Alongside her husband they successfully own a contracting/design company, 40 acre working farm, and a little coffee shop, Willowbrook Grounds in Landis, NC.

She has a heart for people and a love for the Lord that radiates from within. Her lifelong desire was to become a Mama to four children, and through a rugged journey she now holds four in her arms and two little angels forever in her heart.

She's reached lives world wide through her influential instagram @willowbrookfarmlife and her blog Willowbrook Farm Life. Readers are instantly captivated by her easy to read writing style and hilariously funny, true life stories.

She has been featured on podcasts and in Genuine Magazine. Her hope in life is to comfort brokenhearted people and share her love of God with everyone she meets.

Printed in the USA
CPSIA information can be obtained
at www.ICGtesting.com
LVHW062233161123
763958LV00002B/3